Nuclear Medicine Clinical Procedures for Technologists

Nuclear Medicine Clinical Procedures for Technologists

Khalid Jassim

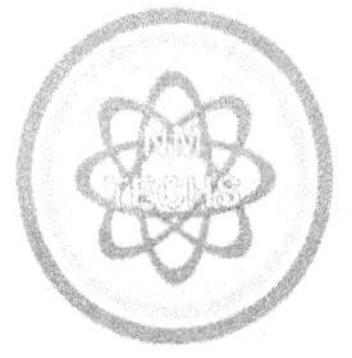

NM Techs™

Educational Recourses for Nuclear Medicine Technologists

DEDICATION

This work is a dedication to The Lady of Heaven.

ladyofheaven.com

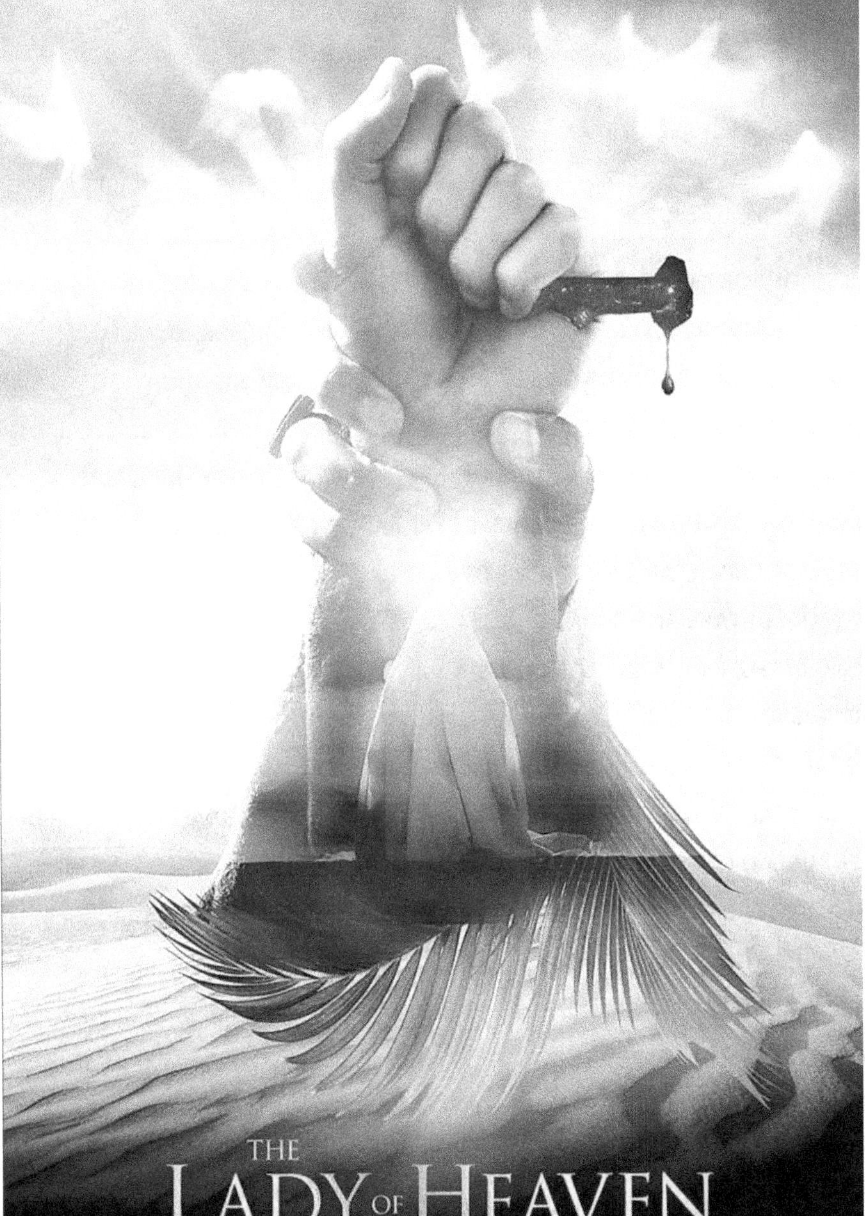
THE
LADY OF HEAVEN
THE UNTOLD STORY

CONTENTS

INTRODUCTION 1

A MESSAGE FOR NUCLEAR MEDICINE STUDENTS 2

CLINICAL TRAINING 3

WHAT INFORMATION SHOULD BE UNDERSTOOD FOR EACH EXAMINATION? 5

EXAMPLE 7

TYPES OF IMAGES IN NUCLEAR MEDICINE AND WHAT ARE THEIR PARAMETERS 9

WHAT IS THE METHOD OF THE CLINICAL EXAMINATION? 12

THIRD ACADEMIC YEAR / FIRST SEMESTER 15

1-THYROID UPTAKE AND SCAN...18

2-LUNG PERFUSION / VENTILATION SCAN 23

3-BONE SCAN 28

A-RENAL SCAN (RENOGRAM) 35

B-RENAL SCAN WITH ANGIOTENSIN CONVERTING ENZYME INHIBITOR (CAPTOPRIL)...38

C-RENAL SCAN FOR TRANSPLANT EVALUATION (RTX) 39

D-GLOMERULAR FILTRATION RATE (GFR) 42

E-RENAL CORTICAL SCAN (DMSA)...45

THIRD ACADEMIC YEAR / SECOND SEMESTER 50

1-HEPATOBILIARY IMAGING..53

2-GASTROINTESTINAL BLEEDING IMAGING (G.I BLEEDING)...........................57

3-MECKEL'S DIVERTICULUM IMAGING 59

4-CARDIAC GATED BLOOD POOL IMAGING 62

5-PARATHYROID IMAGING...65

6-LIVER AND SPLEEN IMAGING..70

7-LIVER HEMANGIOMA IMAGING 73

8-GALLIUM-67 CITRATE IMAGING- GA-67 (INFLAMMATION 76

FOURTH ACADEMIC YEAR / FIRST SEMESTER 81

1-MYOCARDIAL PERFUSION IMAGING (MPI) 84

2-TESTICULAR IMAGING 89

3-LYMPH IMAGING (UPPER & LOWER EXTREMITIES) 91

4- WHOLE BODY IODINE 131 IMAGING WBI 95

FOURTH ACADEMIC YEAR / SECOND SEMESTER 99

1- (LACRIMAL STUDY) DACRYO SCINTIGRAPHY 103

2- SALIVARY GLAND IMAGING.. 105

REFERENCES 108

Introduction

The book "Nuclear Medicine Clinical Procedures for Technologists" serves as a valuable resource not only for Kuwait University's Faculty of Allied Health nuclear medicine students but also for nuclear medicine technology students worldwide. Its purpose is to assist them in their clinical studies and offers valuable insights, general guidelines, and imaging protocols for a wide range of nuclear medicine examinations, drawing from personal experiences of a nuclear medicine technology student gained at various nuclear medicine departments. Whether you are a student, practitioner, or enthusiast of nuclear medicine, this comprehensive guideline is designed to facilitate the understanding and implementing key procedures in this dynamic and ever-evolving field

A Message for Nuclear Medicine Students

Dear nuclear medicine technology students,

In this guide, I'm attempting to provide you with a brief overview of the subjects you will be studying and the nuclear medicine tests you need to be familiar with for your clinical training. The purpose of this guide is to give you a general overview of your study requirements and is not intended to be the sole source for your clinical training. The protocols for nuclear medicine tests mentioned in this guide are just examples. For writing the required reports and studying for the clinical examination, please refer to the protocols used in the nuclear medicine department where your clinical training is taking place and the university-approved textbooks.

I wish you all the best and success

بسم الله الرحمن الرحيم

اخواني و اخواتي طلاب تكنولوجيا الطب النووي
السلام عليكم و رحمة الله و بركاته

في هذه الدليل احاول ان اعطيكم نبذه بسيطة عن المواد التي سوف يتم دراستها ، و ايضا فحوصات الطب النووي التي يجب عليكم معرفتها لاتمام تدرييكم الاكلينيكي. الغرض من هذا الدليل اعطائكم نبذه عامة عن متطلبات دراستكم و ليس الغرض منه ان يكون مصدر الدراسة الوحيد لتدرييكم الاكلينيكي.

بروتكولات فحوصات الطب النووي المذكورة في هذا الدليل هي مجرد مثال ، و لكتابة الريبورتات المطلوبة منكم و للدراسة للامتحان الاكلينيكي يرجى الرجوع الى بروتكولات فحوصات الطب النووي المستخدمة في قسم الطب النووي الذي يجري به تدرييكم الاكلينيكي و الى الكتب الدراسية المعتمدة لدى الجامعة.

مع تمنياتي لكم بالتوفيق و النجاح،،،

Clinical training

Clinical training sets itself apart from typical university courses as it involves students being placed in one of the nuclear medicine departments. For third-year students, this happens over three days a week, and for fourth-year students, it extends to four days a week. The purpose is to provide practical training in various nuclear medicine tests. The standard working hours are from 7:30-8:00 AM to 12:45 PM.

Your training will be supervised by a Certified Instructor (CI), who is responsible for your training and answering all your clinical questions and inquiries. They also oversee your practical examination. Typically, the learning process for nuclear medicine examination involves observing the CI first as they perform the complete examination. Then, students perform the examination with the assistance and supervision of the CI until they have mastered all the steps of the examination. Therefore, I advise students to pay close attention to the CI when conducting the examination, recording all the steps, and also monitor other students when they are performing the examination for learning.

What are the things required for students to know in clinical training?

1. Performing nuclear medicine tests.
2. Image processing.
3. Daily quality control (QC) procedures.
4. Additionally, preparing radioactive materials for patient use, specifically for fourth-year students.

التدريب الاكلينيكي

يختلف التدريب الاكلينيكي عن مواد الجامعة الاخري بانه يتم توزيعكم في احد اقسام الطب النووي لثلاثة ايام في الاسبوع لطلبة السنة الثالثة و اربعة ايام لطلبة السنة الرابعة للتدرب العملي على فحوصات الطب النووي المختلفة. يكون الدوام عادة من الساعة 7:30 الى الساعة 12:45. يتولى الاشراف على تدريبكم مدرب معتمد و هو يكون مسئول عن تدريبكم و الاجابة عن كافة اسئلتكم و استفساركم الاكلينيكية و كذلك يتولى الاشراف على امتحانكم العملي.

طريقة تعلم عمل فحص الطب النووي تكون عادة بمراقبة المدرب أولا و هو يقوم بهذا الفحص كاملا ، و ثم يقوم الطلبة بعمل الفحص بمساعدة و اشراف المدرب حتى يصل الطلبة لدرجة اتقان كافة خطوات الفحص. لذا انصح الطلبة بمراقبة المدرب جيدا عند عمل الفحص و تسجيل كافة الخطوات ، و كذلك مراقبة الطلبة الاخرين عند قيامهم بالفحص للتعلم.

ما هي الاشياء المطلوب من الطالب معرفتها في التدريب الاكلينيكي؟

- عمل فحوصات الطب النووي.
- معالجة الصور.
- عمل فحص الجودة اليومي.
- بالاضافة الى تحضير المادة المشعة للمريض لطلبة السنة الدراسية الرابعة.

What information should be understood for each examination?

- Examination **Name**: Study name
- Examinations Reasons and clinical symptoms: Indications
- Factors that may prevent the examination: Contraindication
- Patient Guidelines before and after the examination: Patient preparation
- Utilized Radiopharmaceutical: Radiopharmaceutical
- The Captured Images and their Parameters: Views & their parameters specific for each image
- Processing and printing the captured images: Image processing

ما هي الأشياء المطلوب معر فتها لكل فحص ؟

- أسم الفحص.
- سبب أجراء الفحص.
- الأمور التي تعارض أجراء الفحص.
- تعليمات و تحضيرات المريض قبل، أثناء، و بعد الفحص.
- المادة المشعة المستخدمة للفحص.
- طرق معالجة و طباعة صور الفحص.

Example

VQ (Lung perfusion) study
- General Indications for lung scans:
  - common clinical indications: Diagnosis of pulmonary embolism
  - Less common clinical indications
    - Document the degree of resolution of pulmonary embolism.
    - Quantify differential pulmonary function before pulmonary surgery for lung cancer
    - Evaluate lung transplants
    - Evaluate congenital heart or lung disease such as cardiac shunts, pulmonary arterial stenoses, and arteriovenous fistulae and their treatment
    - Confirm the presence of Broncho pleural fistula
    - Evaluate chronic pulmonary parenchymal disorders such as cystic fibrosis.
    - Evaluate the cause of pulmonary hypertension
    - Contraindication: Patient should remove any attenuating materials.
- Patient preparation:
  - No specific patient preparation is required.
  - A recent chest x-ray (within 24 hours) should be available for reference. This is adequate for patients who have no changes in signs or symptoms.
  - A more recent chest x-ray (preferably within 1 hour) is necessary in patients whose signs and symptoms are changing.

Tc-99m MAA Lung Perfusion
- Radiopharmaceutical:
  - Tc-99m MAA (macro aggregated albumin)
  - T: 6 hours-140 KeV
  - Dose:
  - Adult: 40-150 MBq (1-4 mCi)
  - Pediatric: 0.74-3.0 MBq / k * g
  - Minimum dose: 7.4 MBq

- o Route of administration: I.V. injection over 3-5 respiratory cycles after asking the patient to cough and take several deep breaths.
- Equipment: gamma camera
- Collimator: LEHR
- Window: 20% centered @ 140 kev
- Patient position: supine or sitting if the patient cannot be supine
- Field of view: Thorax-show both lungs
- imaging time: once injected
- Views:
  - o 1-Anterior/Posterior:
    - Type: static
    - Matrix: 256 x 256
    - Zoom: 1
  - o 2-Right Anterior oblique/ Left posterior oblique:
    - Type: static
    - Matrix: 256 x 256
    - Zoom: 1
  - o 3-Left Anterior oblique/ Right posterior oblique:
    - Type: static
    - Matrix: 256 x 256
    - Zoom: 1
  - o 4-Right lateral/ Left lateral
    - Type: static
    - Matrix: 256 x 256
    - Zoom: 1
- Data processing:
  - o Use the XELERIS software to preview he following images:
  - o Perfusion images:
    - ANT / POST
    - RAO / LPO
    - LAO / RPO
    - RL / LL

Types of images in nuclear
medicine and what are
their parameters.

ما هي انواع الصور في الطب النووي
و ما هي مواصفاتها ؟

In nuclear medicine, there are various types of images obtained using a Gamma Camera, each with specific parameters. The common types of nuclear medicine images include:

Static (planar images)
Parameters:

- MATRIX (64x64, 128x128, 256x256)
- Zoom (1, 1.23...)
- Detector used (detector one, detector two, both detectors)
- Detector angle (0, 45, 90, 180, 360).
- Patient orientation (supine/prone, feet first/ head first)
- Image taken by time or by counts or both whatever come first.

Whole body (wb)

- Total body acquisition, continues static image.

Parameters:

- MATRIX (256X1024)
- Zoom (1)
- Detector used (both detectors)
- Table Speed (8, 10, 12, … cm/min)
- Patient orientation (supine/prone, feet first/ head first)

Dynamic

- A sequence of static images (a series of frames)

Parameters:

- MATRIX (64x64, 128x128)
- Zoom (1, 1.23, …)
- Detector used (detector one, detector two, both detectors)
- Detector angle (0, 45, 90, 180, 360)
- Patient orientation (supine/prone, feet first/ head first)
- Number of Frames
- Time per Frame

Gated

- In gated images an EKG is used to synchronize the acquired frames with the cardiac cycle. Also there is respiratory gating where is frames is synchronized with respiratory cycle.

Parameters:
- Number of Frames
- Center
- Width %
- Forward/backward by third (on/off)
- auto center primary window (on/off)
- auto tracking (on/off)
- Reject PVC Beats (on/off)
- beats to reject post
- PVC threshold

TOMO (SPECT)

- The two detectors circulate around the patient to produce a 3D image.

TOMO Parameters:
- Zoom (1, 1.23, …)
- Orbit (Non circular (body contour) / circular)
- Mode (step & shoot / continuous)
- Number of Views
- Time per View
- Rotation(cw/ccw) clock wise, anti-clock wise
- Starting Angel (0 degree)

TOMO-CT (SPECT-CT)

- A 3D image combined with CT

CT Parameters:
- Scan Type (Helical/ axial)
- Voltage (Kev)
- Current (mA)
- Slice Thickness (1.5… mm)

What is the method of the clinical examination?

Typically, at the end of each rotation, the practical examination is conducted, which is divided into two parts: practical and theoretical.

The Practical Part:

Students are given a patient file, and it is the student's responsibility to read the file, call the patient, ensure the patient follows the examination instructions, explain the examination procedures to the patient, perform the examination on the patient, process the examination images, and print them.

The Theoretical Part:

After completing the practical part, students are asked a series of questions related to the examination they conducted, the daily QC performed in the department, and questions about radiation protection methods.

ما هي طريقة الأمتحان العملي؟

يتم اجراء الامنحان العملي عادة عند نهاية كل فترة تدريب عملي. ينقسم الامتحان الى قسمين عملي و نظري

الجزء العملي:

يتم اعطاء الطالب ملف المريض و يجب على الطالب قراءة الملف و مناداة المريض و التاكد من اتباعه لتعليمات الفحص ، و ثم شرح اجراءات الفحص له ، و ثم اجراء الفحص للمريض و معالجة صور الفحص و طباعتها.

الجزء النظري:

عند الانتهاء من الجزء العملي يتم سؤال الطالب مجموعة من الأسئلة التي تختص بفحص الجودة اليومي الذي يتم عمله في القسم و فحص الطب النووي الذي عمله الطالب و اسئلة عن طرق الحماية من الاشعاع.

مثال على اسئلة الجزء النظري:

Examples of theoretical exam questions:

- What are the daily QC procedures conducted in the department, and why are they performed (peaking, extrinsic, intrinsic, COR, etc.)?
- What type of study did you perform?
- What are the indications for the study?
- What are the contraindications for the study?
- What is the patient preparation procedure?
- What radiopharmaceutical was used?
- What views were taken, and what were their parameters?
- Questions about Image Processing
- What measures are taken to ensure radiation safety for yourself and others?

السنة الدراسية الثالثة

الكورس الأول

The first semester of the third academic year

Third Academic Year / First Semester

The subjects to be studied in this semester:
Digital Imaging and Processing Techniques
In this course, students will study digital images and methods of processing them. This subject is generally straightforward and is studied alongside radiology students.
Medical Radiation Physics 1
This subject is relatively easier than the introductory medical physics course studied in the second year, as its topics are specific to radiology and nuclear medicine.
Nuclear Medicine Chemistry
This subject is divided into theoretical and practical (laboratory) sections. In the laboratory, experiments are conducted, and students are required to prepare reports on these experiments. The practical examination is based on one of these experiments, and in the theoretical section, topics such as chemical equations are covered in the mid-term exam, and in the final exam, theoretical subjects like proteins, and more. This subject is generally straightforward and is studied by second-year medical laboratory students.
Imaging Procedures 1
The Imaging Procedures course is of utmost importance for nuclear medicine students. It covers the theoretical aspects of nuclear medicine examinations in the third academic year, first semester. Examinations of bones, lungs, thyroid glands, and kidneys are covered in this semester, while other examinations are covered in subsequent courses. It is crucial to study this subject through the instructor's explanations and the course textbook. The practical aspect of the examinations studied in the clinical setting will be covered separately.
Clinical 1
This course covers the practical aspect of the examinations studied in the Imaging Procedures course. Students are assigned to undergo practical training in one of the nuclear medicine departments, where they perform practical examinations in nuclear medicine. A clinical exam is conducted for students in one of the examinations they have been trained on in the nuclear medicine department. Clinical training is highly significant for
nuclear medicine students as it qualifies and prepares them for their professional careers in nuclear medicine.

السنة الدراسية الثالثة / الكورس الأول

المواد التي سيتم دراستها في هذا الكورس:

تقنيات تصوير رقمي

يتم في مادة الديجيتال دراسة الصور الرقمية و طرق تحسينها. المادة بشكل عام سهلة و يتم دراستها مع طلبة الاشعة.

فيزياء الاشعاع الطبي 1

هذه المادة في رأيي اسهل من مادة مقدمة في الفيزياء الطبية التي تم دراستها في السنة الثانية ، لان مواضيعها خاصة بالاشعة و الطب النووي.

كيمياء طب نووي + مختبر

مادة كيمياء طب نووي تتقسم الى قسم نظري و قسم عملي (مختبر). في المختبر يتم عمل تجربة و من ثم على الطلبة عمل تقرير عن هذه التجربة و يكون الامتحان العملي في احد هذه التجارب على كافة الطلبة. في القسم النظري يتم دراسة في كمية الميدترم معادلات كيميائية و في كمية الفاينل مواضيع نظرية كالبروتينات و .... ، المادة بشكل عام سهلة و يتم دراستها مع طلبة المختبرات الطبية سنة ثانية.

طرق تصوير اشعاعي 1

مادة البروسيجر هي اهم مادة لطلبة الطب النووي ، و يتم بها الدراسة النظرية لفحوصات الطب النووي. في السنة الدراسية الثالثة الكورس الاول يتم دراسة فحوصات (العظام ، الرئتين ، الغدة الدرقية و الكلى) و في باقي الكورسات يتم تغطية الفحوصات الاخرى. يجب الحرص على دراسة هذه المادة من شرح دكتور المادة بالأضافة الى كتاب المادة. يتم تغطية الجزء العملي للفحوصات التي يتم دراستها في الكلينيكال.

كلينيكال 1

يتم في هذه المادة تغطية الجزء العملي للفحوصات التي يتم دراستها في مادة البروسيجر. حيث يتم توزيع الطلبة للدراسة العملية في احد اقسام الطب النووي للدراسة العملية لفحوصات الطب النووي و يتم اجراء اختبار عملي للطلبة في احدى الفحوصات التي تم التدرب عليها في قسم الطب النووي. الدراسة العملية الكلينيكال مهمة جدا لطلبة الطب النووي حيث انها تؤهلهم و تهيئهم لحياتهم العملية في الطب النووي.

فحوصات الطب النووي

**Third Academic Year /
First Semester
Nuclear Medicine
Examinations**

1. Thyroid Uptake and Scan
2. Lung Perfusion / Ventilation Scan
3. Bone Scan
4. Renal Imaging
    a. Renal Scan (Reno gram)
    b. Renal Scan with Angiotensin Converting Enzyme Inhibitor (Captopril)
    c. Renal Scan for Transplant Evaluation (RTX)
    d. Glomerular Filtration Rate (GFR)
    e. Renal Cortical Scan (DMSA)

Note: The nuclear medicine examination protocols mentioned in this guide are for illustrative purposes only. Please refer to the specific nuclear medicine department for the actual examination protocols in use.

تنويه: بروتكولات فحوصات الطب النووي المذكورة في هذا الدليل هي مجرد مثال توضيحي ، لذا يرجى الرجوع الى بروتكولات فحوصات الطب النووي المستخدمة في قسم الطب النووي الخاص بكم.

1-Thyroid Uptake and Scan

Indications:

detect and localize hyperthyroidism (lose weight-staring gaze) or hypothyroidism (gain weight)
detect and localize metastases for thyroid cancer
differentiation of benign from malignant nodules
post thyroid surgery-Evaluation of thyroid anatomy

Contraindication:

allergy to iodine if it is used
pregnant and breast feeding ladies

Patient preparation:

overnight fasting until 2 hrs. post i-131 ingestion
stop any thyroid medications: thyroxin (T4) for 4-6 weeks- and Cytomel (T3) for 2 weeks
should not take (thyroid blocking agent) for 5 days before study
avoid eating iodine containing food. (cabbage-turnips-greens-soy beans-shellfish-seafood-kelp-large amount of table salt)

Thyroid Uptake

Radiopharmaceutical:

Radiopharmaceutical	T 1/2	Dose	ADULT DOSE	target	Route of administration
I-131 (sodium iodine)	8 days - 364 Kev	10uci-13uci	10 uCi	thyroid	131I capsule Oral (PO)

Equipment:

Equipment		uptake probe
	Collimator	flat field
	Window	20% centered @ 364 Kev
	Patient position	supine or sitting position - probe anterior
	Field of view	neck and lower 2/3 of thigh
	imaging time	2 hours and 24 hours
	distance from probe	about 25 cm

Procedure steps:

I-131 -4hr and 24hr	
1-standard capsule measurements	a- place I-131 capsule in the (neck phantom) and place the probe perpendicular to the phantom and scan for (1 min)
	b- remove the capsule from the phantom and measure room background by scanning the empty phantom with the probe for (1 min)
2-patient measurements	a- position the probe over patient lower 2/3 of thigh and scan for (1 min)
	b- position the probe over patient neck and scan for (1 min)

Thyroid Scan

Radiopharmaceutical:

Radiopharmaceutical	T 1/2	Dose	ADULT DOSE	critical organ	Route of administration
Tc-99m pertechnetate	6 hours- 140 Kev	2-10 mci	5 mCi	Thyroid	I.V. injection
Localization	Active transport. 99mTcO4 – trapped but not organified. Iodine organified by thyroid and held in cells or follicular lumen.				

Equipment:

Equipment	Camera	gamma
	Collimator	pinhole , (or LEHR)
	Window	20% centered @ 140 Kev
	Patient position	supine- chin up-pillow under shoulder
	Field of view	neck fully (extended)
	Camera	anteriorly
	imaging time	15-20 min after injection

Views & their parameters:

Views	matrix	zoom	time	count	
1-Full syringe	256x256	2.67	1 min		
2-Empty syringe	256x256	2.67	1 min		
3- Neck image	256x256	2.67	5 min	150 Kcount	thyroid gland fits two thirds of field of view
4- Neck image with marker	256x256	2.67	1 min		Co-57 marker on substernal notch
5-LAO (left anterior oblique)	256x256	2.67	5 min	150 Kcount	
6-RAO (right anterior oblique)	256x256	2.67	5	150	

Image processing:

For processing thyroid images, follow these steps:[1]

1. Statics:
   - Load all static images.
   - Annotate the static images as necessary.

Thyroid Uptake scan, processing steps:

1. Select the following images:
   - Pre and post-syringe images.
   - Anterior (thyroid) image.
   - Injection site image if it was taken.
2. Choose the "thyroid uptake index" protocol.
3. Define the thyroid Region of Interest (ROI):
   - Create the thyroid ROI manually by double-clicking and drawing the ROI around the thyroid.
4. Proceed with the review.
5. Print the inverse image.

---

[1] Image processing software used (GE Healthcare Xeleris)

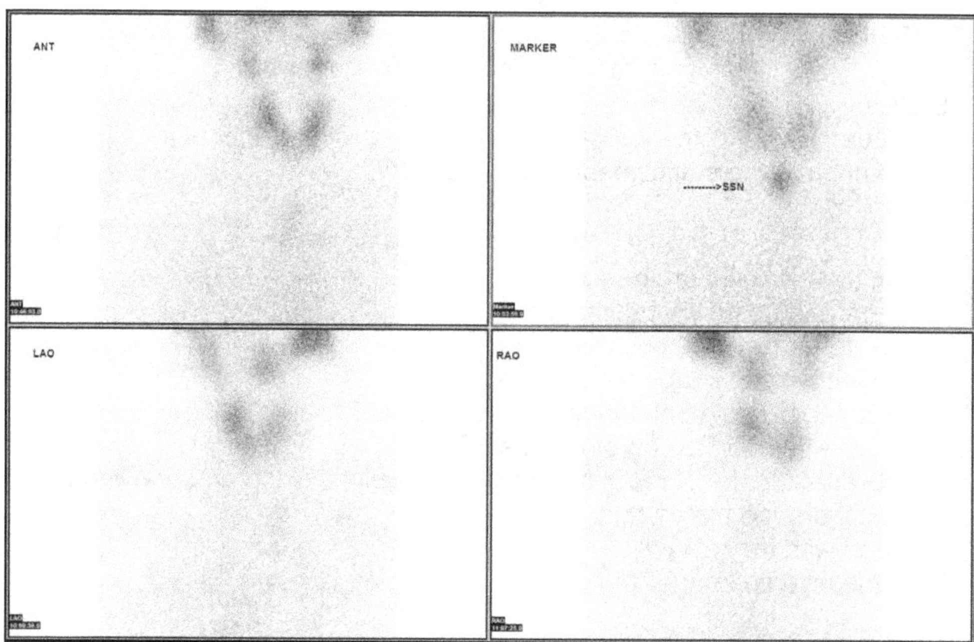

Figure 1 Thyroid static images

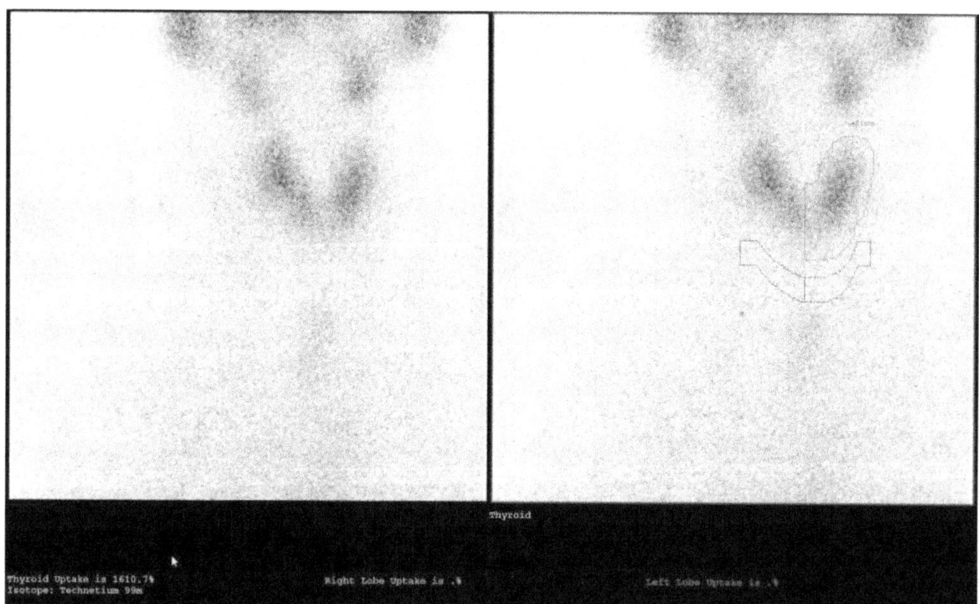

Figure 2 Thyroid uptake images

2-Lung Perfusion / Ventilation Scan

Indications

common clinical indications : Diagnosis of pulmonary embolism
Less common clinical indications:
1.chest pain.
2.shortness of breath
3.Evaluate lung transplants
4. Evaluate congenital heart or lung disease such as cardiac shunts, pulmonary arterial stenosis, and arteriovenous fistulae and their treatment
5. Confirm the presence of Broncho pleural fistula
6. Evaluate chronic pulmonary parenchymal disorders such as cystic fibrosis.

Contraindication:

contraindication	pregnant and breast feeding ladies (given low dose if necessary)
	Right to left shunts (unless it is the reason for the scan)
	not be performed on patients with pulmonary hypertension

Patient preparation:

Patient preparation	No specific patient preparation is required.
	A recent chest x-ray (within 24 hours) should be available for reference. This is adequate for patients who have no changes in signs or symptoms.
	A more recent chest x-ray (preferably within 1 hour) is necessary in patients whose signs and symptoms are changing.

A- Tc-99m MAA Lung Perfusion:

Radiopharmaceutical:

Radiopharmaceutical	T 1/2	Dose	Route of administration	ADULT DOSE
Tc-99m MAA - (macro aggregated albumin)	6 hours- 140 Kev	5 mCi	I.V. injection over 3-5 respiratory cycles after asking the patient to cough and take several deep breaths.	5 mci
Localization	Blood flow to pulmonary capillary			

B- Technegas Lung Ventilation:

Radiopharmaceutical:

Radiopharmaceutical	T 1/2	Dose	Route of administration
Technegas-(Tc-99m-labeled carbon)	6 hrs	10-15 mCi	Inhalation (by a mouthpiece or tight fitting mask)

Equipment:

Camera	Collimator	Window	Patient position	Field of view
Gamma	LEHR	20%	supine or sitting if the patient cannot be supine	Chest

Views & their parameters:

- The same images are taken for both perfusion and ventilation.

1	type	matrix	zoom	count-Kcount	notes
	static	256x256	1	500	detector 1+2
STATIC	1-ANT/POST				
	2-RAO/LPO-45 degree				
	3-R LAT / L LAT-90 degree				
	4-RPO/LAO-135 degree				

2	collimator	LEHR
SPECT	matrix	128*128
	zoom	1
	number of view	60 (120 total)
	time per view	15sec
	degree of rotation	180 (180 for each detector total 360)
	start angle	0
	detector configuration	180 (180 for each detector total 360)
	orbit	Non circular
	mode	step & shoot
	rotation	ccw
	body contour	on

	scan type	Helical
CT	Voltage	120 kV
	Current	20 mA
	Slice thickness	5 mm
	pitch	12
	direction	cranial-caudal
	SDOV	large
	CTDI VOL	1.51mGY
	DLP	37 mGy.cm
	care dose / SMART	0-on
	scan time	4.7 sec
	delay	3 sec
	rotation time	.6 sec
	use for	AC
	number of images	41
	matrix	512
	CT RANGE	Partial

Image processing:

For V/Q (Ventilation/Perfusion) imaging, follow these steps:[2]

Statics:

- Load all static images.
- Annotate the images for different views, such as Ant PERF, POST, RLAT, RAO, LPO, L LAT, LAO, and RPO.

SPECT-CT:

- Select TOMO image.
- Choose the appropriate CT image, with 1.25 mm slice thickness, or 2.5mm.
- Proceed with "Volimitrix."
- If there is no motion in the images, choose "original."
- If there is motion, select "auto," and then proceed to select "corrected" for further processing.

---

[2] Image processing software used (GE Healthcare Xeleris)

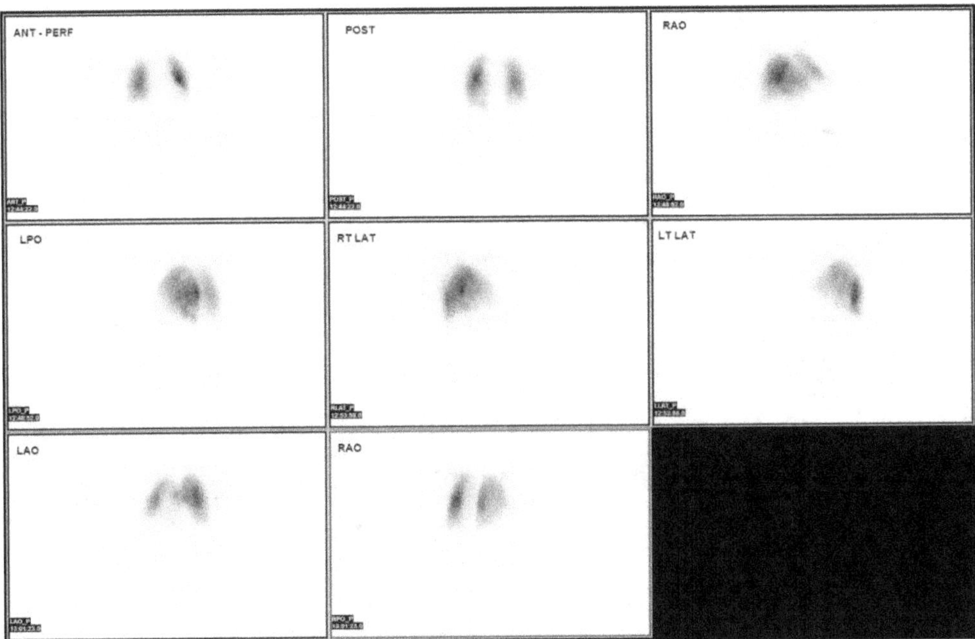

Figure 3 Lung Perfusion Static images

3-Bone Scan

Indications

Indications	malignancy: skeletal metastases detection and follow up
	stress fracture
	differentiation between osteomyelitis and cellulitis
	occult fractures
	prosthesis evaluation for infection or loosening
	avascular necrosis

Contraindication:

contraindication	pregnant and breast feeding ladies

Patient preparation:

Patient preparation	Hydration and void before exam
	remove metal objects

Radiopharmaceutical:

Radiopharmaceutical	T 1/2	Dose	Route of administration	ADULT DOSE
Tc-99m MDP or HDP	6 hours- 140 Kev	20-30 mCi	I.V	20 mCi
hydroxy-methelene diphosphonate				
Localization	Chemisorption			

Views & their parameters:

1	type	matrix	zoom	time
DYNAMIC flow	dynamic	128x128	1	2 or 3 min
	60 frames-3 seconds each- total 3 min **or**			
	40 frames-3 seconds each- total 2 min			

2	type	matrix	zoom	time	notes
STATIC bp	static	256x256	1	3 min	by time 3min, and count, which come first, use 2 detectors
	blood pool-tissue phase , same position as flow				
	(pelvis, spine, chest) -700-1000 kcount				
	(skull, thigh, knee) -500-600 kcount				
	rest 150-300 kcount				

Static Images that can be taken:

- Feet: internal rotation-external rotation-planter
- Knee: anterior/posterior - lateral with shield between knees & knee raised
- Skull: anterior/posterior - vertex
- Shoulder: anterior/posterior + heart covered with shield
- TOD (tail on detector) for pelvis & bladder
- Frog position for head of femur

3	type	matrix	zoom	notes
WB	static	256x1024	1	time depend on patient height
	speed to 17-20 cm/min			
	scan the whole patient body start from head to feet			

Patient instruction	drink lot of water before the second scan (delay scan) to clear the tracer from the body
	void to decrease the bladder exposure to radiation
	the radiotracer concentrated on the bone after 10-30 min of injection, so blood pool images should be done in less than 10 min after injection to avoid showing the bone
	the 2-3 hours delay to clear the background

- After 2-4hrs (delay scan) the same views is repeated again (statics and WB)

- A SPECT-CT may be required:

SPECT		
	collimator	LEHR
	matrix	128*128
	zoom	1
	number of view	60
	time per view	15-20 sec
	degree of rotation	180 (180 for each detector total 360)
	start angle	0
	detector configuration	180 (180 for each detector total 360)
	orbit	Non circular
	mode	step & shoot
	rotation	cw

CT		
	scan type	Helical
	Voltage	120 kV
	Current	20 mA- **SMART MA/care dose**
	Slice thickness	2.5mm
	pitch	12
	direction	cranial-caudal
	care dose / SMART	0-on
	use for	AC
	number of images	41
	matrix	512

Image processing:

Nuclear medicine bone scan image processing steps:[3]

- Flow Image:
    - reframe by 3, anterior & posterior images.
    - select (flow ant or flow post), then load to new, and choose the image tab to reframe.
    - write '3' in the output field, then apply & quit.
    - clear the original (old) image by selecting file-clear.
    - format the reformatted image: select screen format, scroll tab, press the up arrow to display all frames.
    - choose 5x4 layout.
    - annotate as (ant 9 sec/frame dynamic or post 9 second/frame dynamic).
- Whole Body Image:
    - load to new (whole body early & delay).
    - annotate as (ant whole body blood pool, post whole body blood pool, ant whole body delay, post whole body delay).
    - Static Images:
    - load all static images to new.
    - annotate for each image, specifying ant, post, right, left, early, delay, and mention body part name.
- Tomographic CT (TOMO CT) images:
    - Select TOMO image.
    - Choose the appropriate CT image, with 1.25 mm slice thickness, or 2.5mm.
    - Proceed with "Volimitrix."
    - If there is no motion in the images, choose "original."
    - If there is motion, select "auto," and then proceed to select "corrected" for further processing.

---

[3] Image processing software used (GE Healthcare Xeleris)

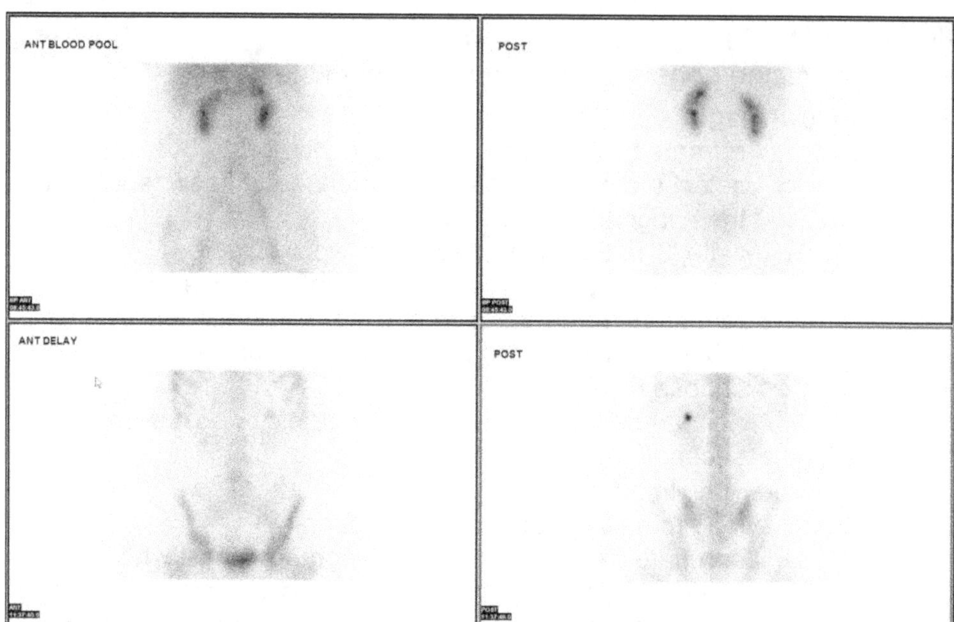

Figure 4 Bone static images

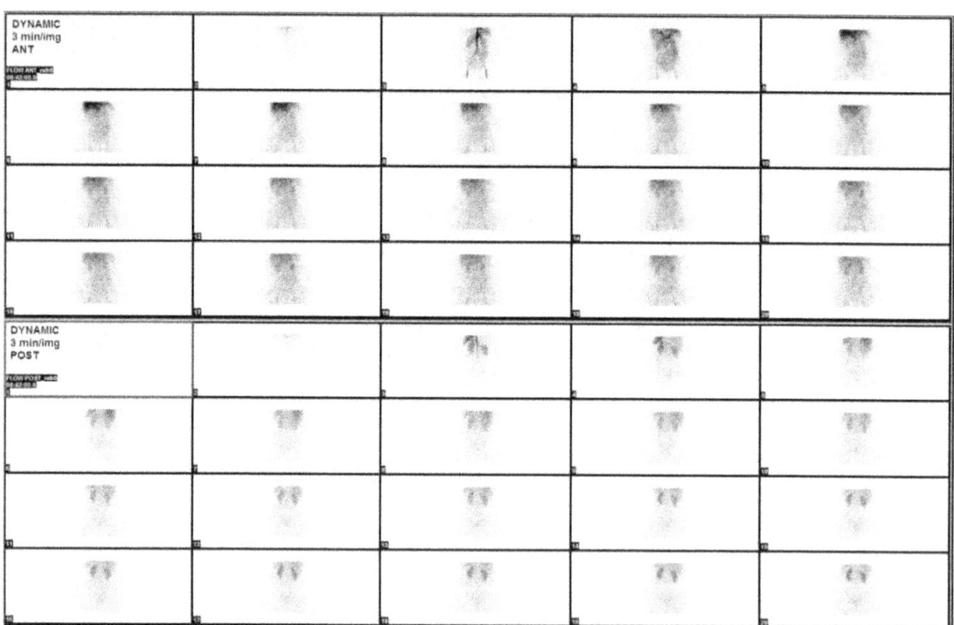

Figure 5 Bone dynamic images

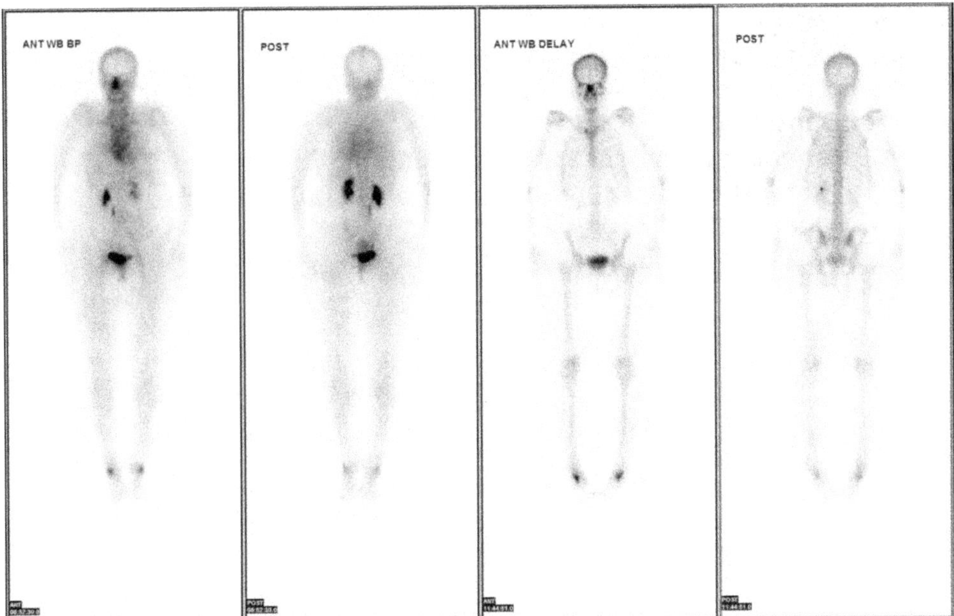

Figure 6 Bone whole body images

4-Renal Imaging
   a) **Renal Scan (Renogram)**
   b) **Renal Scan with Angiotensin Converting Enzyme Inhibitor (Captopril)**
   c) **Renal Scan for Transplant Evaluation (RTX)**
   d) **Glomerular Filtration Rate (GFR)**
   e) **Renal Cortical Scan (DMSA)**

A-Renal Scan (Renogram)

Indications

Indications	blood flow -routine renal function
	Evaluation of renal perfusion and function
	Detection and evaluation of urinary tract obstruction -UTO/-PUJO-pelvic ureter junction obstruction
	Evaluation of etiology of renal failure

Contraindication:

contraindication	pregnant and breast feeding ladies
	2-3 weeks after-contrast study

Patient preparation:

Patient preparation	remove all attenuating objects
	hydrated (drink 500 ml water) and void before scan

Radiopharmaceutical:

Radiopharmaceutical	T 1/2	Dose	Route of administration	critical organ
TC-99m MAG-3	6 hours-140 Kev	5-10 mci	I.V injection	kidney
MAG-3: mercapto acetyl tri-glycine				

Views & their parameters:

	type	matrix	zoom	time	notes
1-dynamic	Dynamic	128*128	1.23	21 min	detector 2 (posterior)
	show kidneys and bladder				
	Zoom can be changed depending on patient (adult: 1.23- pediatric:2)				
	30 frame-for 2 sec each-total 1 min				
	120 frame-for 10 sec each-total 20 min				

	type	matrix	zoom	time	notes
2-Pre void	static	128*128	1.23	2 min	Taken if Bladder is Cut

	type	matrix	zoom	time	notes
3-post void	static	128*128	1.23	2 min	Taken after Patient void

- Extra post void delay maybe ordered.

Image processing:

Renal image processing steps:[4]
Renal Analysis:

- Select (flow & post void) images and choose the Renal Analysis protocol.
- Specify the parameters:
    - Number of kidneys:2 kidneys,
    - Radiopharmaceutical used: MAG3,
    - camera-based clearance: NONE,
    - pediatric state (yes/no)
    - diuretic used (yes/no)
- Draw ROIs on the right and left kidneys on the function image.
- Draw ROIs on the background of the right and left kidneys on the function image.
- Select the aorta and move the mouse over it in the image.
- Proceed to Clinical Summary.
- For motion in dynamic images, apply motion correction if needed.

Dynamic images reframe:

- Select (flow & post void) images and load to a new workspace.
- Reframe the flow image in (phase 2) by 12.

---

[4] Image processing software used (GE Healthcare Xeleris)

- Clear the old image.
- Choose an appropriate screen format.
- Annotate the images as needed.

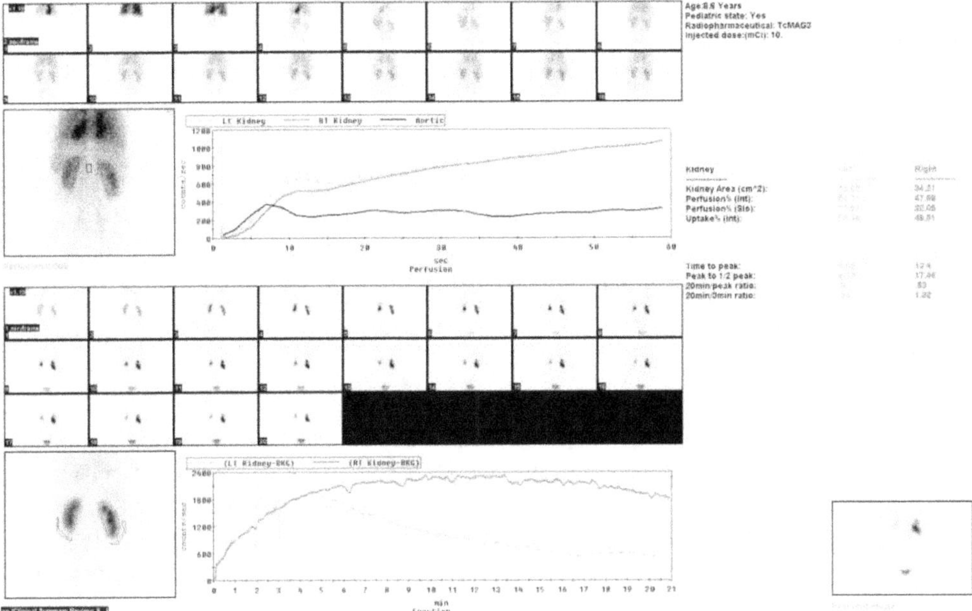

Figure 7 Renal analysis

B-Renal Scan with Angiotensin Converting Enzyme Inhibitor (Captopril)

Indications

- Diagnosis of Reno vascular hypertension

Patient preparation:

Patient preparation	stop all ACE (captopril) inhibitors -2-3 days
	stop diuretics- which lead to dehydration
	give Lasix which increase clearance
	hydrated (drink 500 ml water) and void before scan

The procedures of this exam is similar to renal scan, except that in this one before the exam starts, the patient is administered an Angiotensin-converting enzyme inhibitor such as Captopril. After that, the patient blood pressure is measured four times every fifteen minutes. If the blood pressure was normal, the patient is injected with 99mTc-MAG3 and normal renal imaging protocol is done.

C-Renal Scan for Transplant Evaluation (RTX)

Indications

- Evaluation of renal transplant

Contraindication:

contraindication	pregnant and breast feeding ladies
	2-3 weeks after-contrast study

Patient preparation:

Patient preparation	remove all attenuating objects
	hydrated (drink 500 ml water) and void before scan

Radiopharmaceutical:

Radiopharmaceutical	T 1/2	Dose	Route of administration	critical organ
TC-99m MAG-3	6 hours-140 Kev	5-10 mci	I.V injection	kidney

MAG-3: mercapto acetyl tri-glycine

Views & their parameters:

	type	matrix	zoom	time	notes
1-dynamic	Dynamic	128*128	1.23	21 min	detector 1 only (anterior)
	show Transplant kidneys				
	start once doctor inject				
	30 frame-for 2 sec each-total 1 min				
	120 frame-for 10 sec each-total 20 min				

2-post void	type	matrix	zoom	time	notes
	static	128*128	1.23	2 min	Taken after Pt void (if Pt able to Void)

Image processing:

RTX renal image processing steps:[5]

Renal Analysis for Transplant Kidney:

- Select (flow & post void) images and choose the Renal Analysis protocol.
- Specify the parameters:
    - Number of kidneys: transplant kidneys,
    - Radiopharmaceutical used: MAG3,
    - camera-based clearance: NONE,
    - pediatric state (yes/no)
    - diuretic used (yes/no)
- Draw an ROI on the kidney in the function image.
- Draw ROI for background on both function and perfusion images.
- Select iliac and move the mouse over it in the image.
- Adjust the perfusion index by aligning vertical white lines at the start and peak of perfusion.
- Proceed to Clinical Summary.

---

[5] Image processing software used (GE Healthcare Xeleris)

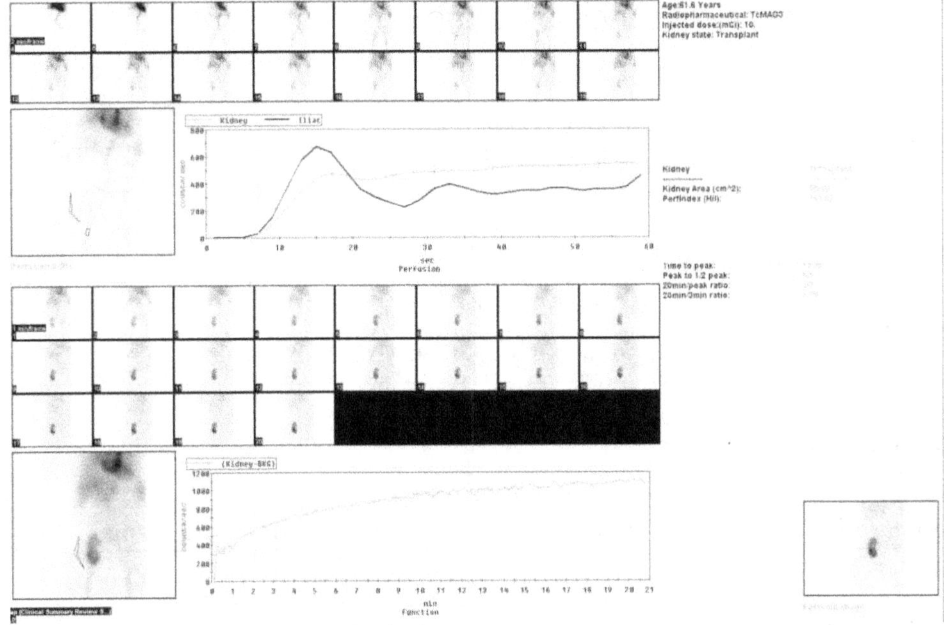

Figure 8 Renal transplant image Analysis

D-Glomerular Filtration Rate (GFR)

Indications

Indications	prospect kidney donor
	Evaluation of glomerular filtration rate

Contraindication:

contraindication	pregnant and breast feeding ladies
	2-3 weeks after-contrast study

Patient preparation:

Patient preparation	remove all attenuating objects
	hydrated (drink 1000 ml water) and void before scan

Radiopharmaceutical:

Radiopharmaceutical	T 1/2	Dose	Route of administration
TC-99m DTPA	6 hours- 140 Kev	5-10 mci	I.V injection

DTPA:di-ethylene tri-amine penta acetic acid

Views & their parameters:

1-full syringe	type	matrix	zoom	time	notes
	static	128*128	1.23	30 sec	detector 2 only (posterior)

2-DTPA dynamic	type	matrix	zoom	time	notes
	Dynamic	128*128	1.23	21 min	detector 2 only (posterior)
	show kidneys and part of bladder				
	1-1 min image for 2 sec for 30 frame				
	2- 20 min image 15 sec for 80 frame				

3-empty syringe-(post syringe)	type	matrix	zoom	time	notes
	static	128*128	1.23	30 sec	detector 2 only (posterior)

4-post void	type	matrix	zoom	time	notes
	static	128*128	1.23	2 min	detector 2 only (posterior)

5- injection site	type	matrix	zoom	time	notes
	static	128*128	1.23	30 sec	detector 2 only (posterior)
	after removing the canola				
	place the injection site on detector 2 and scan for 30 sec				
	after finish instruct patient to not to:(smoke- drink caffeine- eat chocolate)				
	the patient should come back to take sample blood 3 times 2 hours after injection , 3 hours after injection and 4 hours after injection)				

Image processing:

GFR (Glomerular Filtration Rate) image processing steps:[6]

- Renal Analysis for GFR Calculation:
- Select all relevant images (pre & post syringe, flow & post void, injection site) and choose the Renal Analysis protocol.
- Specify the parameters:
  - Number of kidneys: 2 kidneys,
  - Radiopharmaceutical used: DTPA,
  - camera-based clearance: Gates,
  - pediatric state (yes/no)
  - diuretic used (yes/no)

---

[6] Image processing software used (GE Healthcare Xeleris)

- Draw ROIs on both the right and left kidneys in the function image.
- Draw ROIs on the background of both the right and left kidneys in the function image.
- Select the aorta and move the mouse over it.
- Proceed to Camera-Based Clearance.
- Proceed to Clinical Summary.

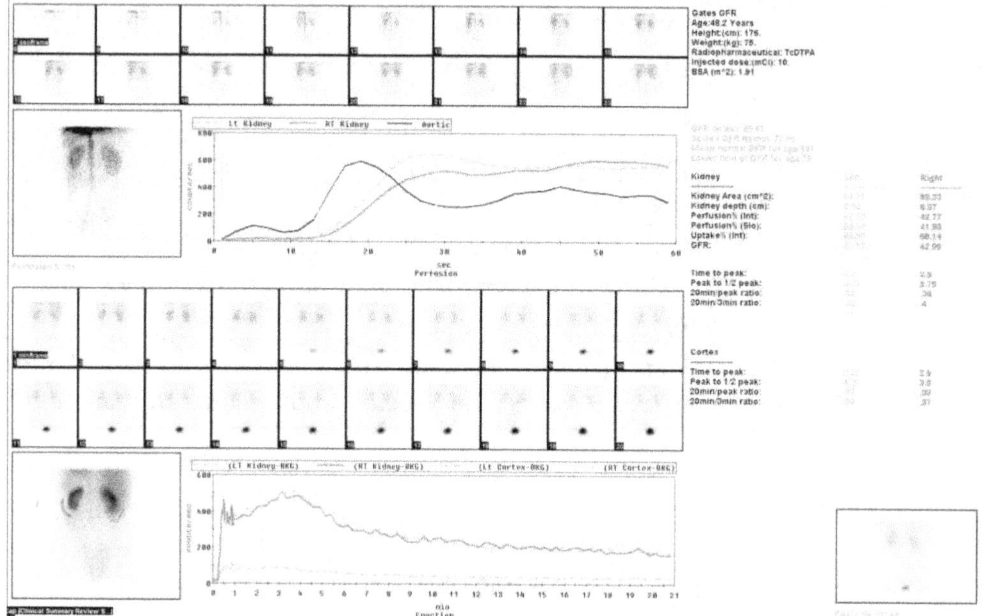

Figure 9 Image analysis for GFR study

E-Renal Cortical Scan (DMSA)

Indications

Indications	Evaluation of renal trauma
	Evaluation of Kidney shape-size-site
	UTI-urinary tract infection
	scarring
	pyelonephritis-infection- reflux

Contraindication:

contraindication	pregnant and breast feeding ladies
	2-3 weeks after-contrast study

Patient preparation:

Patient preparation	remove all attenuating objects
	scan will be 2 to 3 hours after injection patient should be hydrated and void before scan

Radiopharmaceutical:

Radiopharmaceutical	T 1/2	Dose	Route of administration	critical organ
TC-99m DMSA	6 hours- 140 Kev	1-5 mci	I.V injection	kidney
DMSA: die-mercapto succinic acid				

Views & their parameters:

Statics	type	matrix	zoom	time	count-Kcount	notes
	static	256*256	1-2	about 15min	500 kcount	detector 1 and 2
1- Ant/Post	10 min or 500 kcount					
2-RAO/LPO	10 min or 500 kcount - 45 degree					
3-LAO/RPO	10 min or 500 kcount- 315 degree					

Tomo		
	collimator	LEHR
	matrix	128*128
	zoom	1-1.6
	number of view	60
	time per view	20 sec
	degree of rotation	180 (180 for each detector total 360)
	start angle	0
	detector configuration	180 (180 for each detector total 360)
	orbit	Non circular
	mode	step & shoot
	rotation	cw
	body contour	on

Image processing:

DMSA (Dimercaptosuccinic Acid) image processing steps:[7]

- DMSA Analysis:
    - select only (ant, post) image and choose the dmsa protocol.
    - enter patient information (age, h&w), and click ok.
    - define rois for kidneys and their backgrounds:
    - select left post button, draw roi on left post kidney, then click on left post background button.
    - select right post button, draw roi on right post kidney, then click on right post background button.
    - select left ant button, draw roi on left ant kidney, then click on left ant background button.
    - select right ant button, draw roi on right ant kidney, then click on right ant background button.
    - proceed to basic data.
- Static Images:
    - Select all static images and load to new for DMSA.
    - Annotate static images (Ant, Post, RAO, LAO, RPO, LPO)
    - Tome (if applicable):
    - Select TOMO, then Volimitrix.
    - if there's no motion, select original.
    - if there is motion, select auto, then select corrected.

---

[7] Image processing software used (GE Healthcare Xeleris)

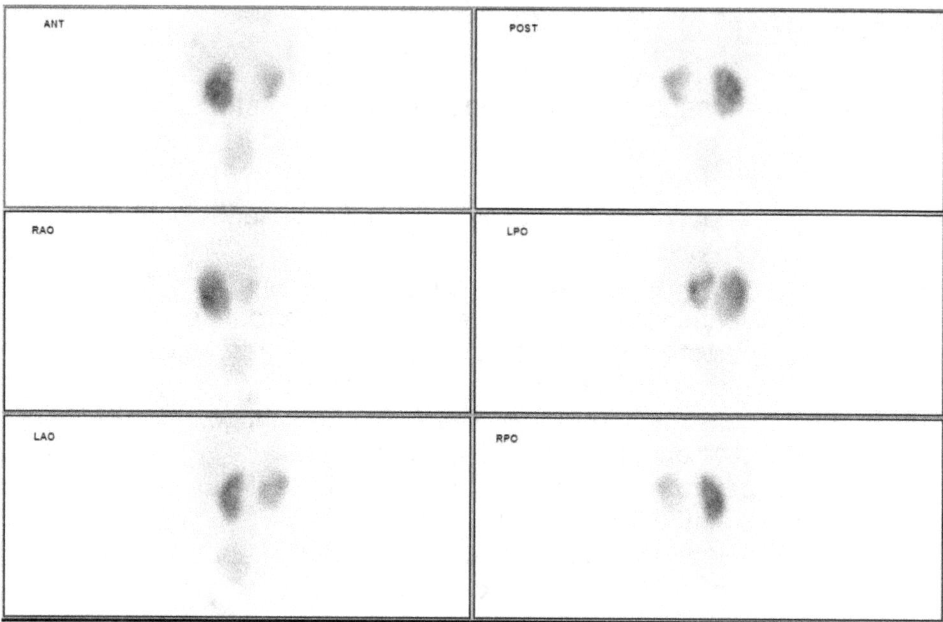

Figure 10 DMSA static images

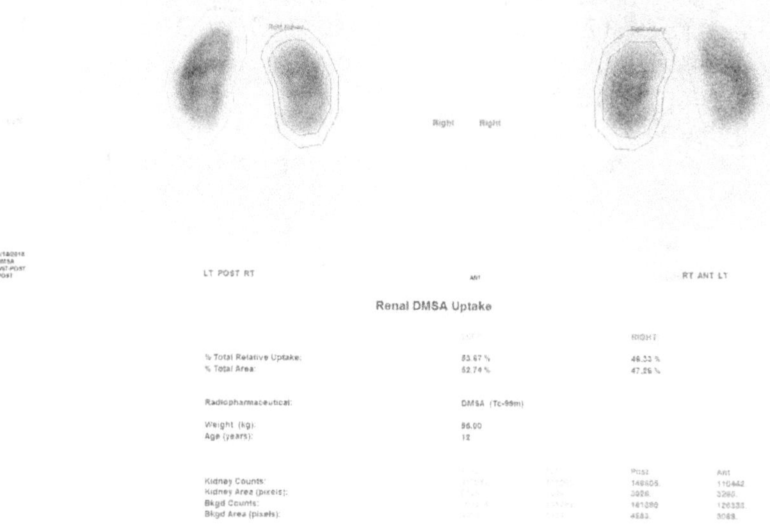

Figure 11 DMSA analysis

The second semester of the third academic year

السنة الدراسية الثالثة
الكورس الثاني

Third Academic Year / Second Semester

The subjects that will be studied in this semester are:

1. Radiation Protection & Radiobiology
In this subject, the risks of ionizing radiation and methods of protection from it are studied.

2. Pathology in Imaging
In this subject, various diseases are studied in a general manner.

3. Medical Radiation Physics 2
Most the subject has a focus on nuclear medicine topics. It is not studied with radiology students, but there are common topics studied together.

4. Imaging Procedures 2
In the third academic year, second semester, the following nuclear medicine examinations are studied:
- Hepatobiliary
- Gastrointestinal Bleeding
- Meckel's Diverticulum
- Gated Blood Pool
- Parathyroid
- Spleen
- Liver Hemangioma
- Adrenal Gland
- Ga-67

5. Clinical (2)
This subject covers the practical part of the examinations studied in the Procedures subject in the first and second semesters of the third academic year. The practical exam includes all the examinations studied in the first and second semesters.

السنة الدراسية الثالثة / الكورس الثاني

المواد التي سيتم دراستها في هذا الكورس:

الوقاية من الاشعاع و بيولوجيا الاشعاع
في هذه المادة يتم دراسة مخاطر الاشعة المؤينة و طرق الوقاية منها.

1علم الامراض التصويري
في هذه المادة يتم دراسة الأمراض بشكل عام، غالبا تكون كمية الميدتيرم مكثفة ، لكن الفاينل يكون اقل كثافة.

فيزياء الاشعاع الطبي 2
معظم كمية هذه المادة خاصة بمواضيع في الطب النووي لذا لا يتم دراستها مع طلبة الأشعة و لكن يوجد مواضيع مشتركة يتم دراستها معهم.

طرق تصوير اشعاعي 2
في السنة الدراسية الثالثة الكورس الثاني يتم دراسة الفحوصات التالية:
Hepatobiliary, G.I Bleeding, Meckel's' diverticulum, Gated blood pool, parathyroid, spleen, Liver hemangioma, Adrenal gland, Ga-67

كلينيكال 2
يتم في هذه المادة تغطية الجزء العملي للفحوصات التي يتم دراستها في مادة البروسيجر في السنة الدراسية الثالثة الكورس الأول بالأضافة الى الكورس الثاني. أي ان الامتحان العملي يشمل كافة الفحوصات التي تم دراستها في الكورس الأول و الثاني.

Third Academic Year / Second Semester Nuclear Medicine Examinations

السنة الدراسية الثالثة / الكورس الثاني

فحوصات الطب النووي

1. Hepatobiliary Imaging
2. Gastrointestinal Bleeding Imaging (G.I Bleeding)
3. Meckel's' diverticulum Imaging
4. Cardiac Gated blood pool imaging
5. Parathyroid Imaging
6. Liver and Spleen Imaging
7. Liver hemangioma Imaging
8. Gallium-67 Citrate Imaging- Ga-67 (Inflammation)

Note: The nuclear medicine examination protocols mentioned in this guide are for illustrative purposes only. Please refer to the specific nuclear medicine department for the actual examination protocols in use.

تنويه: بروتكولات فحوصات الطب النووي المذكورة في هذا الدليل هي مجرد مثال توضيحي ، لذا يرجى الرجوع الى بروتكولات فحوصات الطب النووي المستخدمة في قسم الطب النووي الخاص بكم.

1-Hepatobiliary Imaging

Indications

Indications	cholecystitis
	acute (calculous or acalculous)
	inflammation of gallbladder (GB)
	cholelithiasis
	abdominal (especially right upper quadrant) pain.
	obstruction
	hepatic transplant
	gallbladder function
	post-gallbladder surgery for suspected leakage

Patient preparation:

Patient preparation	npo 4hrs before study
	infant npo 2hr
	void before scan

Radiopharmaceutical:

Radiopharmaceutical	T 1/2	Dose	Route of administration	ADULT DOSE
HIDA hepatobiliary-(iminodiacetic acid).	6 hours-140 Kev	3–15 mCi	i.v	5 mCi
Localization	Polygonal cell uptake and excretion, follows bile path, IDA agents are removed from the blood stream by hepatocytes using active transport and are excreted into the bile unconjugated.			

- Sometimes a form of CCK is given prior to the injection of the radiotracer to ensure that the gallbladder is clear

Views & their parameters:

1	Type	matrix	zoom	time
Flow	DYNAMIC	128*128	1	1 min
	30 frame- 2 sec per frame-60 sec or 60f/2 sec			
	position to show liver and GB			

2	Type	matrix	zoom	time
DYNAMIC	DYNAMIC	128*128	1	1 Hour
	60 frame- 60 sec per frame-3600sec			

3	type	matrix	zoom	time
STATICS	static	256x256	1	5 min
	1-ANT- 300 sec @ the end of the study			
	2-RLAT- 300 sec-to separate GB from kidney and bowel			
	extra 3-LAO to separate GB from kidney and bowel			

- if GB not shown after 1-hour delay or morphine given to increase bile secretion.

Image processing:

the steps for processing HIDA images:[8]
- Statics:
  - Load the static images to a new workspace.
  - Annotate them. If you have both pre and post-fatty meal images, annotate as (ANT PRE FATTY MEAL, ANT 30 min post FATTY MEAL).
- Dynamic Images:
  - Reframe both ANT and POST dynamic images by 3, with a dynamic of 3 min/IMG.
- Gallbladder Ejection Fraction:

---

[8] Image processing software used (GE Healthcare Xeleris)

- o Select dynamic Images
- o Select Gallbladder Ejection Fraction protocol.
- o Draw ROI over gallbladder, then proceed to review summary.

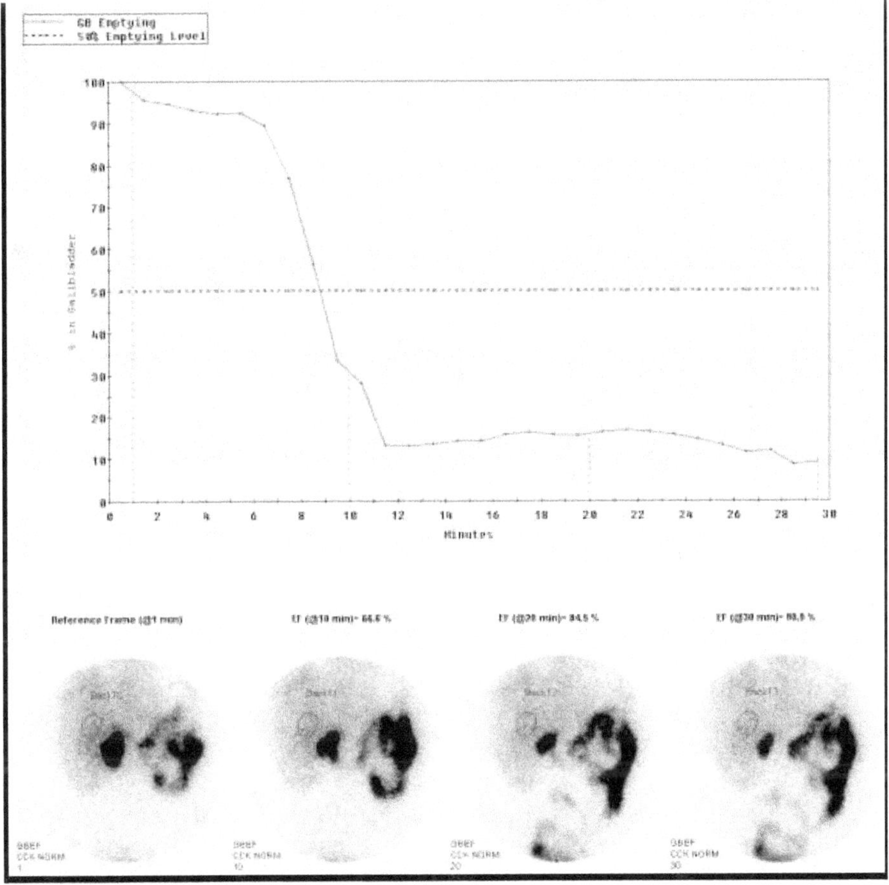

Figure 12 HIDA Reframed GBEF review summary

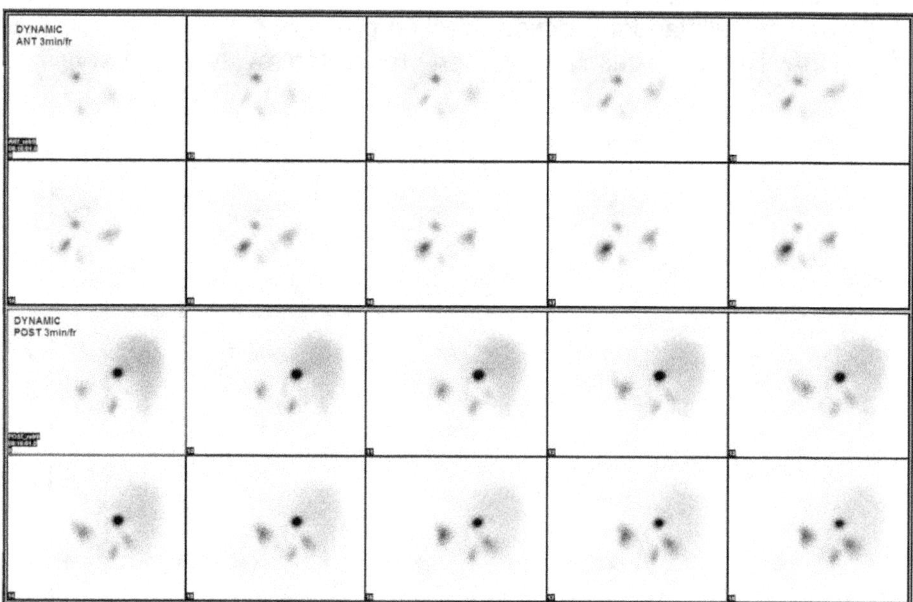

Figure 13 HIDA Reframed dynamic ANT/POST image

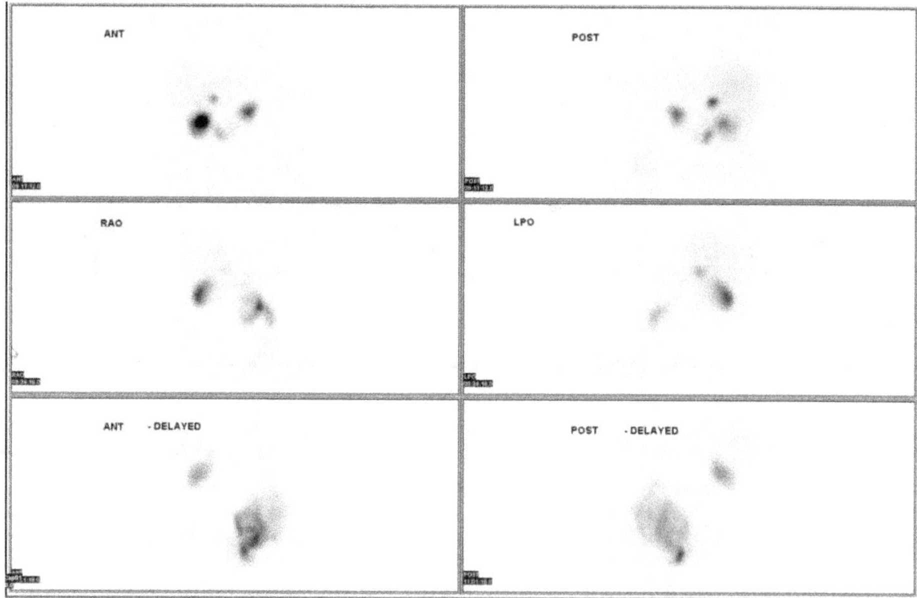

Figure 14HIDA Reframed static images

2-Gastrointestinal Bleeding Imaging (G.I Bleeding)

Indications

Indications	Identify active gastrointestinal bleeding
	Identify non gastrointestinal bleeding

Patient preparation:

- Void before study

Radiopharmaceutical:

Radiopharmaceutical	T 1/2	Dose	Route of administration
Tc99m labeled RBC	6hr, 140 Kev	20-25	i.v
OR Tin COLLOID	6hr, 140 Kev	10	i.v

Views & their parameters:

1	type	matrix	zoom	time
DYNAMIC	Dynamic	128	1	about 1 hours
	1-flow- 40 f / 3 sec 2 min			
	2- 120 f / 30 sec 1hr , for 30 minute if tin colloid used			
	show abdomen and pelvis			
	If tin colloid used dynamic 30 min			

2	type	matrix	zoom	time
Statics	static	256x256	1	5 min
	1-ANT/POST			
	2-RLAT/L LAT			

- Extra View: SPECT-CT

Image processing:

the steps for processing images:[9]

- Static Images:
  - Load to new all static images and Annotate
- Dynamic Images:
  - Reframe both ANT and POST dynamic images by 6

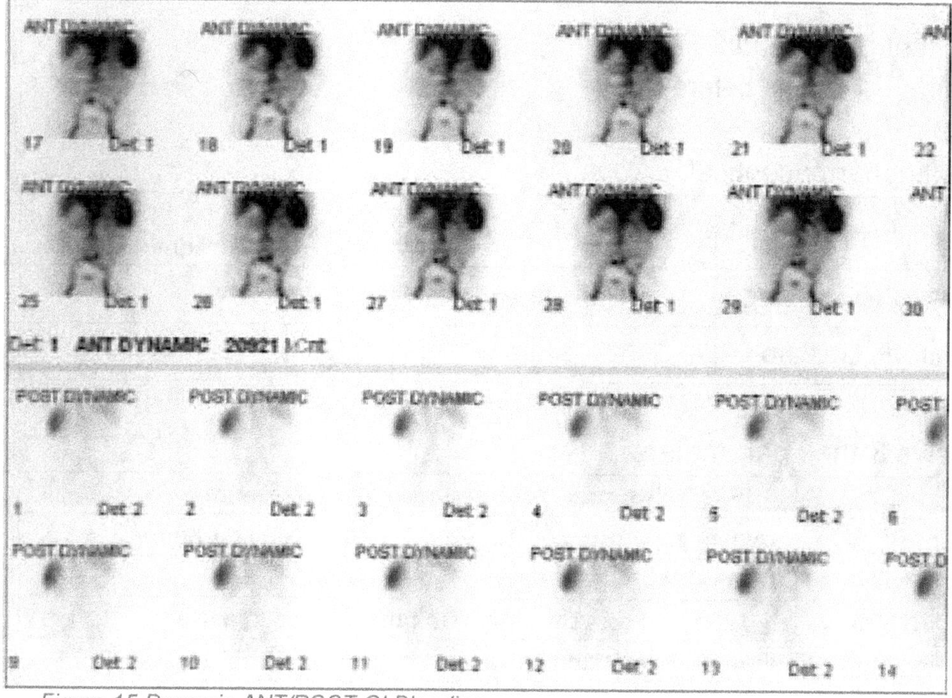

Figure 15 Dynamic ANT/POST GI Bleeding

---

[9] Image processing software used (GE Healthcare Xeleris)

3-Meckel's diverticulum Imaging

Indications

Indications	Localization of a Meckel's diverticulum with functioning gastric mucosa
	gastrointestinal bleeding, ulceration
	abdominal pain

Patient preparation:

Patient preparation	NPO for 4–12 hours. Infants: NPO equal to normal feeding time minus 30 minutes
	discontinue thyroid blocking agents, e.g., perchlorate or saturated solution of potassium iodide 48 hours before study.
	void before, during, after procedure-no barium studies 48 hours before study.
	stop zarontin 2-3 days-

Radiopharmaceutical:

Radiopharmaceutical	T 1/2	Dose	Route of administration	ADULT DOSE
Tc-99m pertechnetate	6 hr, 140 Kev	10–15 mCi	I.V	10 mCi
Localization	Active transport, concentrated and rapidly secreted by the epithelial tissue of the (ectopic) gastric mucosa			

Views & their parameters:

Dynamic	1-flow- 2f/ 60 sec 2 min
	2- 120f / 30 sec 1 hr
	matrix 128x128
	show abdomen and pelvis
EXTRA-delay static or SPECT/CT	

Image processing:

Meckel's image processing steps:[10]

- Dynamic Images:
  - Reframe the images by 3 or 5 for ant and post images based on statics duration (3 min for 3, 5 min for 5).
  - Select (flow ant or flow post), then load to new, and choose the image tab to reframe.
  - In the output field, write either '3' or '5', then apply & quit.
  - Select the original (old) image and clear it by choosing file-clear.
  - Format the reformatted image: Select screen format, scroll tab, and press the up arrow to display all frames.
  - Choose a 5x4 layout.
  - Annotate as (dynamic Ant 3 min/image or dynamic Post 3 min/image) or (dynamic Ant 5 min/image or dynamic Post 5 min/image).
- Static Images:
  - Load all static images to a new workspace.
  - Annotate them as (Ant, Post, RT LAT, LT LAT).

---

[10] Image processing software used (GE Healthcare Xeleris)

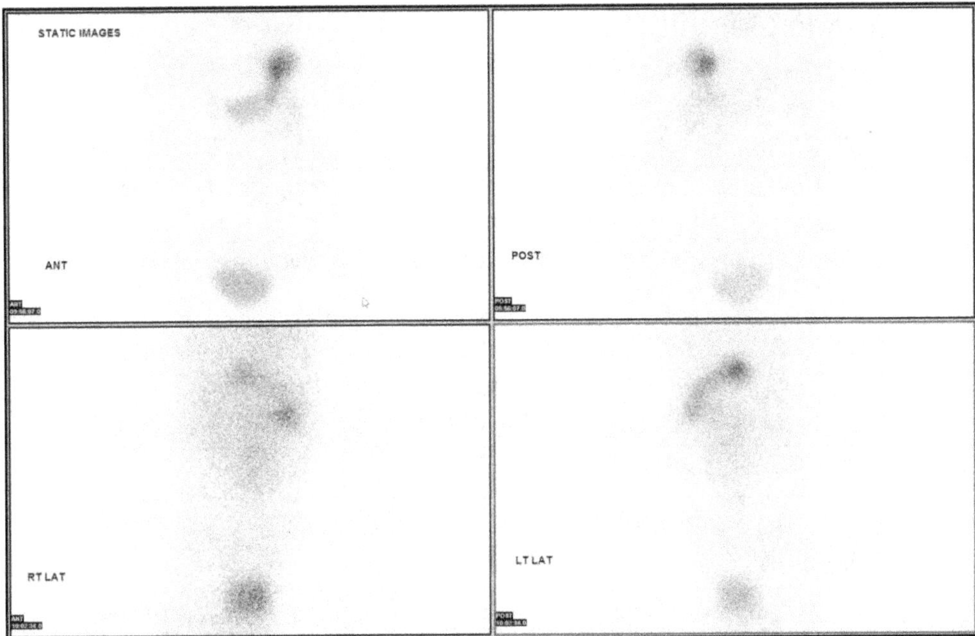

Figure 16 Meckel's diverticulum static images

4-Cardiac Gated blood pool imaging

Indications

Indications	Evaluation of left and sometimes right (for congestive heart failure [CHF]) wall motion.
	Calculation of ejection fraction, ventricular volume, cardiac output, and diastolic function
	coronary artery disease (CAD).
	Evaluation of patient's heart condition before and/or after surgery, chemotherapy, or radiation therapy.
	ischemia & non ischemia

Contraindication:

contraindication	allergic to pyrophosphate or phosphates.-severe arrhythmia
	unstable medical condition.-chest pain.

Patient preparation:

Patient preparation	NPO 4–8 hours-
	discontinue cardiac medications and caffeine ~4 hours before

Radiopharmaceutical:

Radiopharmaceutical	T 1/2	Dose
Tagged red blood cells (RBC) by pyrophosphate (pyp) in combination with 99mTcO4 –(pertechnetate)	6 hours Energies: 140 keV	20–25 mCi
Localization	Compartmental, tagged to, and circulating with blood	

- Patient is injected with PYP
- Hook up three- or five-lead ECG. Check R–R wave.
- after 20 min, he is injected with tcO4, then scan is started

Views & their parameters:

- First Anterior image is done for checking only normal counts.
- If Normal LAO is taken

<table>
<tr><td rowspan="5">LAO</td><td>matrix</td><td>zoom</td><td>width</td><td>counts</td><td>frame</td><td>notes</td></tr>
<tr><td>64*64</td><td>3.2</td><td>30%</td><td>6000</td><td>24</td><td>d1 only</td></tr>
<tr><td colspan="6">LAO ~35–60° looking for best septal wall separation, slight caudal tilt, 5–10%, to camera can help, LLAT, and sometimes RLAT or RAO (looking for "shoe" picture), displaying anterior and inferior wall motion and apex.</td></tr>
<tr><td colspan="6">head out , supine</td></tr>
<tr><td colspan="6">start from 30 degree , then move 2 degrees until best separation</td></tr>
<tr><td colspan="6">caudal tilt may be used to separate LV and L atrium</td></tr>
</table>

Image processing:

Cardiac Gated blood pool image processing:

- select MUGA LAO 45 degree, select MUGA protocol, draw ventricular ROI & calculate ejection fraction

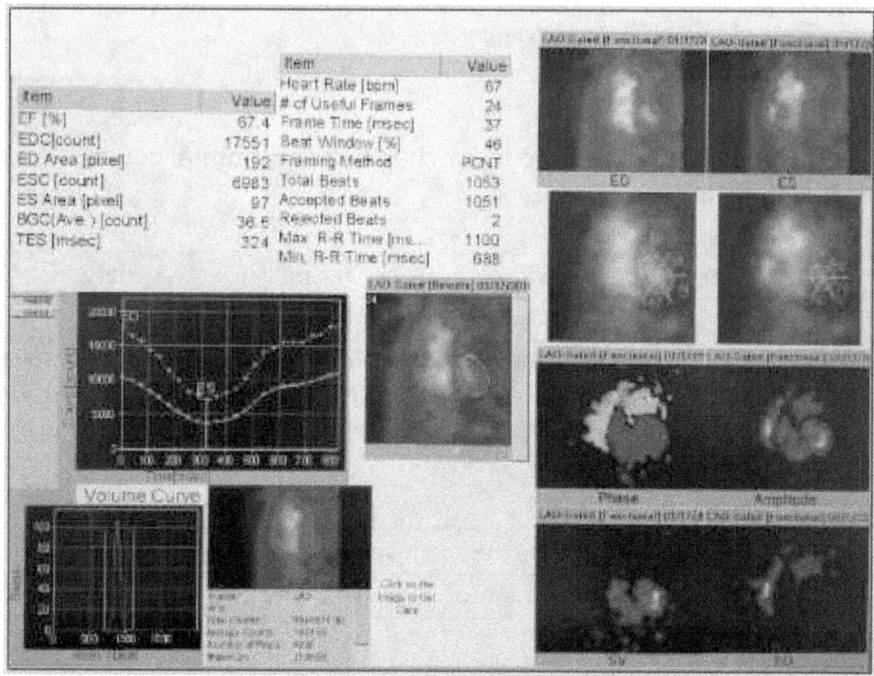

Figure 17 Gated BP image process

5-Parathyroid Imaging

Indications

Indications	parathyroid cancer
	adenomas-localization not detection-before operation

Contraindication:

contraindication	Patient on calcium medications.-
	pregnant and breast feeding ladies

Patient preparation:

Patient preparation	patient should be off thyroid medications for 5 days
	contrast studies 1 week

Radiopharmaceutical:

Radiopharmaceutical	T 1/2	Dose		ADULT DOSE	critical organ
Tc-99m MIBI (sestembi)	6 hours- 140 Kev	MIBI 20-30 mci		25	I.V. injection
Localization	Tc-sestamibi Passive transport in proportion to blood flow into thyroid and normal and abnormal parathyroid tissue, remaining longer in adenomatous and hyperplastic tissue.				

Equipment:

Camera	Collimator	Window	Patient position	Field of view	imaging time
Gamma	LEHR or pinhole	20% centered @ 140 Kev	supine- chin up- pillow under shoulder-head first	neck fully (extended)	5 min after injection

Views & their parameters:

1	type	matrix	zoom	time	Collimator	notes
STATIC 5min	static	256x256	2.57	8 min	LEHR	
	show parathyroid , salivary gland and top of the heart for reference.					

2	type	matrix	zoom	time	Collimator	notes
STATIC 45min	static	256x256	2.57	8 min	LEHR	
	Similar to the 5 min image					

3		
	collimator	LEHR
SPECT @ 45 min	**matrix**	128*128
	zoom	1
	time per view	20 sec
	orbit	Non circular
	mode	step & shoot
	rotation	cw
	body contour	on
CT	**scan type**	Helical
	Voltage	120 kV
	Current	20 mA
	Slice thickness	2.5 mm
	pitch	12
	matrix	512
	CT RANGE	Partial

4	type	matrix	zoom	time	Collimator	notes
STATIC 2hour	static	256x256	2.57	8 min	LEHR	
	Similar to the 5 min image					

- If Subtraction is required the patient come again at least after 24 hours, to be injected with 5 mCi 99m-TC, then after 15 min of injection a static image is taken to be subtracted from the 5 min parathyroid image.

Subtraction	type	matrix	zoom	time	Collimator	notes
Thyroid STATIC 5min	static	256x256	2.57	8 min	LEHR	Image after 15 min of injection
	Similar to the 5 min parathyroid image					

Image processing:
Parathyroid image processing steps:[11]

- Subtraction:
  - Rename (parathyroid-5min image) to (ANT_P) by selecting it, right-clicking, and choosing "Attribute" then "Rename."
  - Rename (Thyroid image) to (ANT_T) in a similar way.
  - Merge the (thyroid & parathyroid) studies by right-clicking and selecting "MERGE."
  - Select (ANT_P & ANT_T) images and choose the parathyroid protocol.
  - Draw a Region of Interest (ROI) on the Parathyroid image.
  - Proceed with Co-Registration and adjust the ROI on Thyroid image.
  - Check (more & less subtraction, smooth & less smooth subtraction) for desired changes.
  - Proceed to Review Summary.
- Static Images:
  - Load all static images to a new workspace.
  - Annotate them as (5 min, 45 min, 2 HR, Thyroid) or (TC_MIBI ANT 5 min, 45 min, 2 HR, TC_PERTEHNITATE ANT).

---

[11] Image processing software used (GE Healthcare Xeleris)

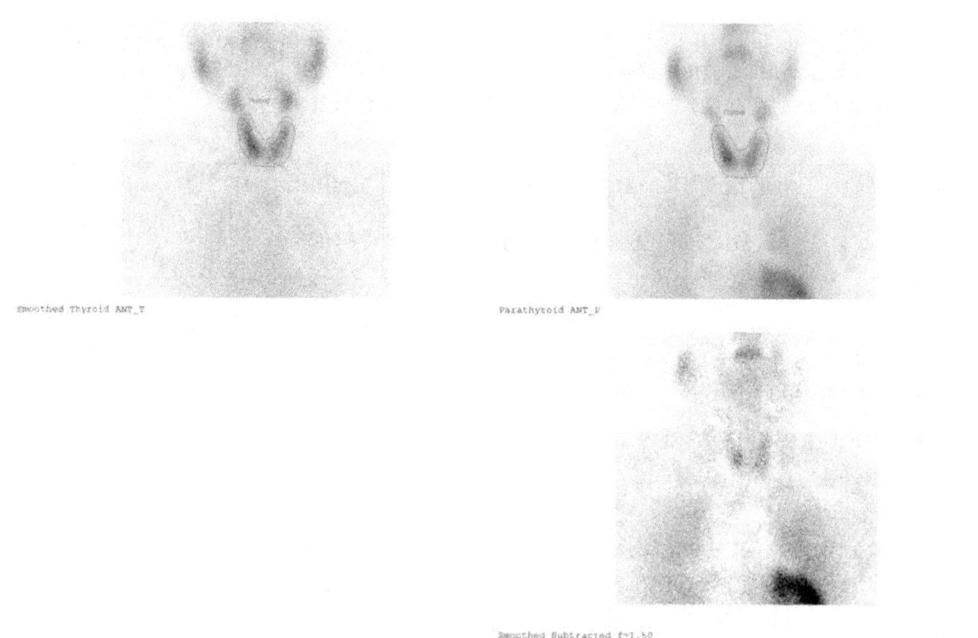

Figure 18 Tc99m & MIBI statics

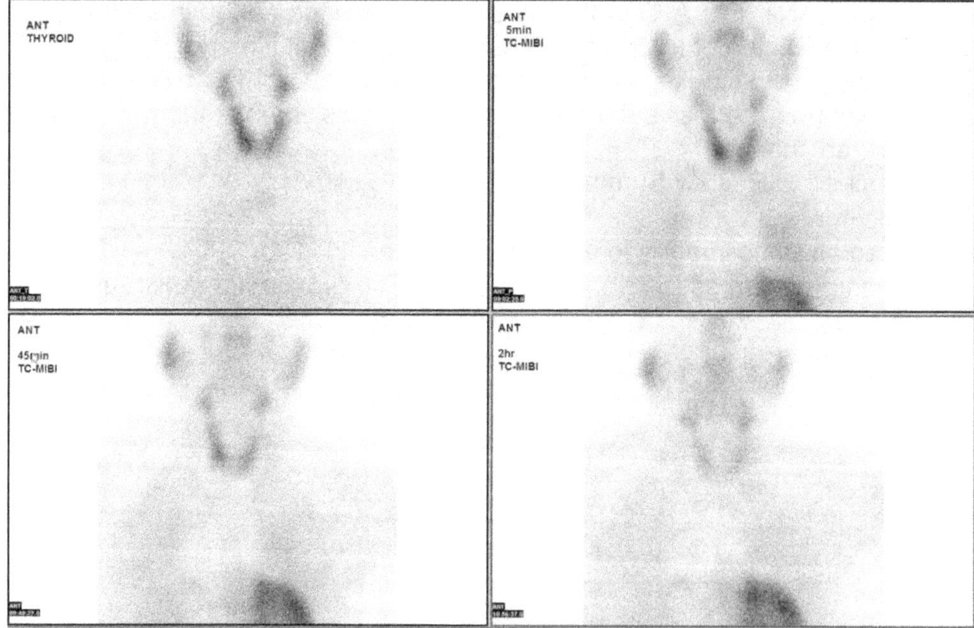

Figure 19 Subtraction Images

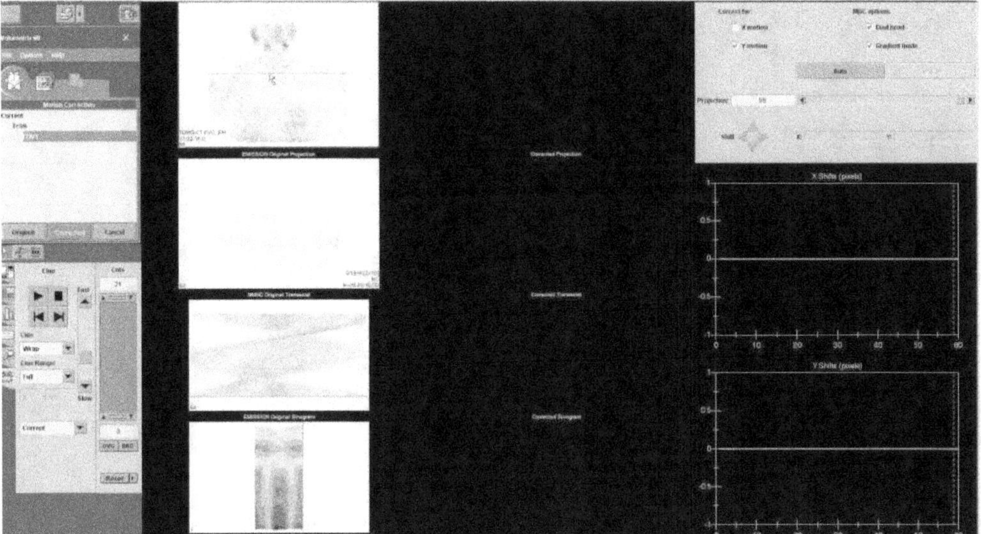

Figure 20 MIBI SPECT-CT

6-Liver and Spleen Imaging

Indications

Indications	Evaluation of Hepatic Function
	Evaluation of liver or spleen size
	Evaluation of liver or spleen focal lesions
	Evaluation of liver or spleen Trauma
	Focal nodular hyperplasia
	Hypersplenism

Radiopharmaceutical:

Radiopharmaceutical	T 1/2	Dose	Route of administration	ADULT DOSE
99m TC-tin colloid	6 hours- 140 Kev	5 mCi	I.V	5 mCi
Localization	Trapping in reticuloendothelial system RES			

Views & their parameters:

	type	matrix	count-Kcount	notes
STATICS	static	256x256	by count 500	both detectors
	show upper abdomen include liver & spleen			
	Image After 5-10 min of injection			
	1-ANT/POST			
	2-RAO/LAO			
	3-RT LAT/ LT LAT			
	4-RPO/LAO			

	type	matrix	zoom	count-Kcount	notes
STATIC-MARKER	static-	256x256	1	by time 10 min	1detector 1
	500 k-counts				
	Marker from xiaphoid parallel to rips				

- Extra: SPECT-CT

Image processing:

Liver & Spleen image processing steps:[12]

- Statics:
  - Load all static images for Anterior (Ant), Posterior (Post), Right Lateral (RT LAT), and Left Lateral (LT LAT) views.
  - Annotate these static images.
- Dynamic Images:
  - Load both and Posterior flow images.
  - Reframe and Annotate Anterior (flow ant 4 sec/image) and Posterior (flow post 4 sec/image) flow images

---

[12] Image processing software used (GE Healthcare Xeleris)

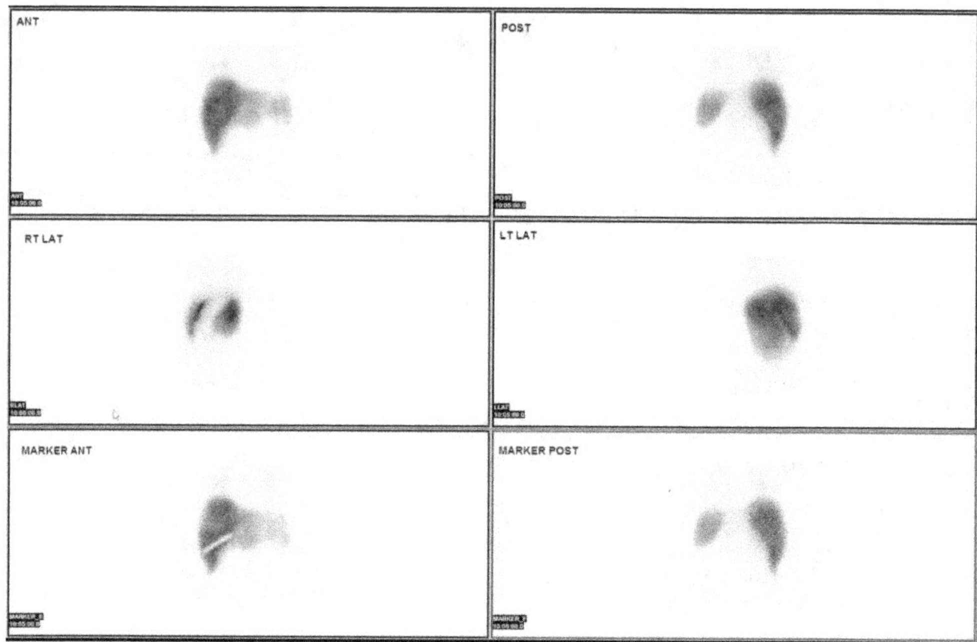

Figure 21 Liver-Spleen static images

7-Liver Hemangioma Imaging

Indications

- To evaluate Liver Hemangioma

Radiopharmaceutical:

Radiopharmaceutical	T 1/2	Dose	Route of administration
Tc99m labeled RBC	6hr, 140 Kev	20-25	i.v

Views & their parameters:

1	type	matrix	zoom	time
	dynamic	128	1	3 min
DYNAMIC	xiaphoid on center- show liver			
	flow: 60 F / 3 sec			

	type	matrix	count-Kcount	notes
	static	256x256	by count 500	both detectors
STATICS	1-ANT/POST			
	2-RAO/LAO			
	3-RT LAT/ LT LAT			
	4-RPO/LAO			

- Extra: SPECT-CT

Image processing:

For processing Hemangioma images, follow these steps:[13]

- Static Images
  - Load all static images for Anterior (Ant), Posterior (Post), Right Anterior Oblique (RAO), Left Anterior Oblique (LAO), Right Lateral (RT LAT), and Left Lateral (LT LAT) views.
  - Annotate the static images accordingly.
- Dynamic Images:
  - Reframe both Anterior (Ant) and Posterior (Post) flow images by a factor of 3, with a dynamic frame rate of 3 min/image.

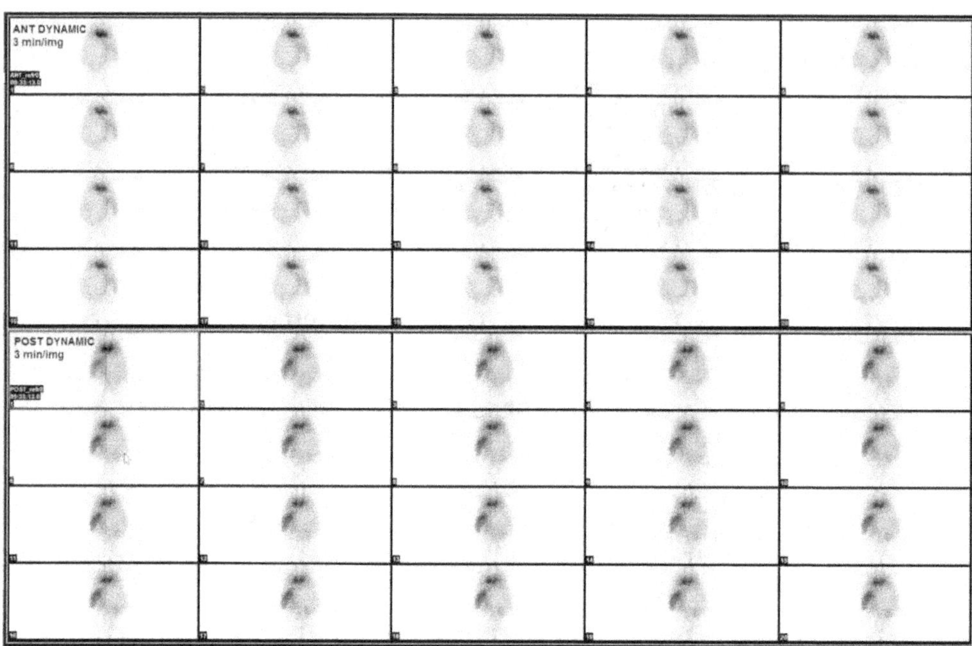

Figure 22 Liver Hemangioma dynamic images

---

[13] Image processing software used (GE Healthcare Xeleris)

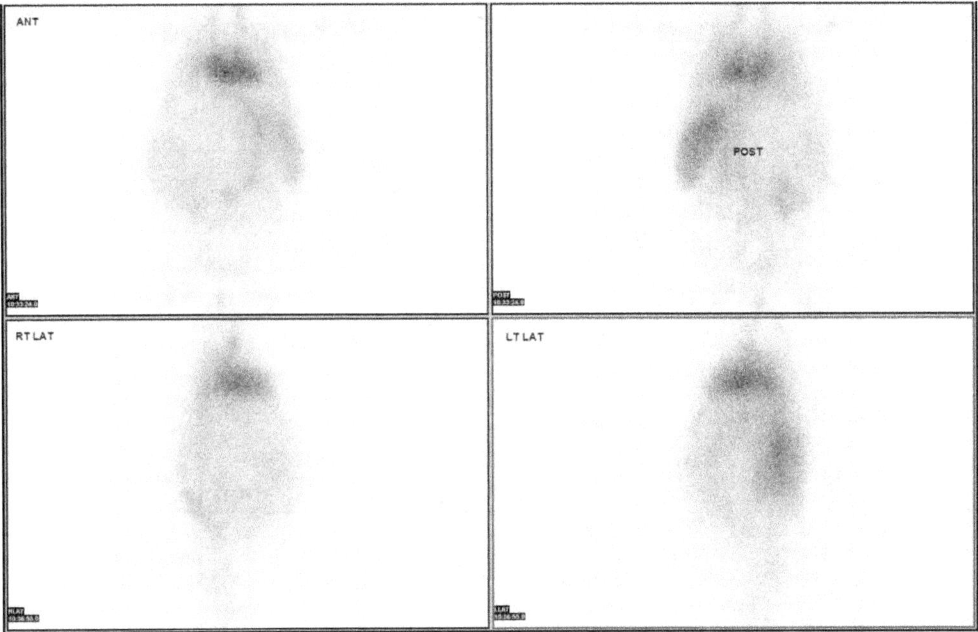

Figure 23 Liver Hemangioma static images

8-Gallium-67 Citrate Imaging- Ga-67 (Inflammation)

Indications

Indications	Fever of unknown origin
	Evaluation of abscesses (chronic inflammation)
	Evaluation of sarcoidosis, tuberculosis (lymphocytic or granulomatous)
	Myocardial or pericardial inflammation

Radiopharmaceutical:

Radiopharmaceutical	T 1/2	Dose	Route of administration	ADULT DOSE
Gallium citrate (Ga-67)	78 hours- 93,185,300,394 Kev	3-6 mCi	I.V	5 mCi
Localization	Iron binding proteins			

Equipment:
- Medium Energy Collimator

Views & their parameters:
- First day patient is injected, imaging at 24, 48, 72 hours

	type	matrix	zoom			
WB	static	256x1024	1			
	speed to 10 cm/min					

	type	matrix	zoom	time	notes
SPOT	static	256	1	5 min	both detectors
	position patient to show abdomen and include liver				

- Extra view: SPECT-CT

Image processing:

Image processing steps:[14]
- Static Images
  - Load all static.
  - Annotate the static images accordingly.
- Whole Body Image:
  - load to new (whole body early & delay).
  - annotate images accordingly.

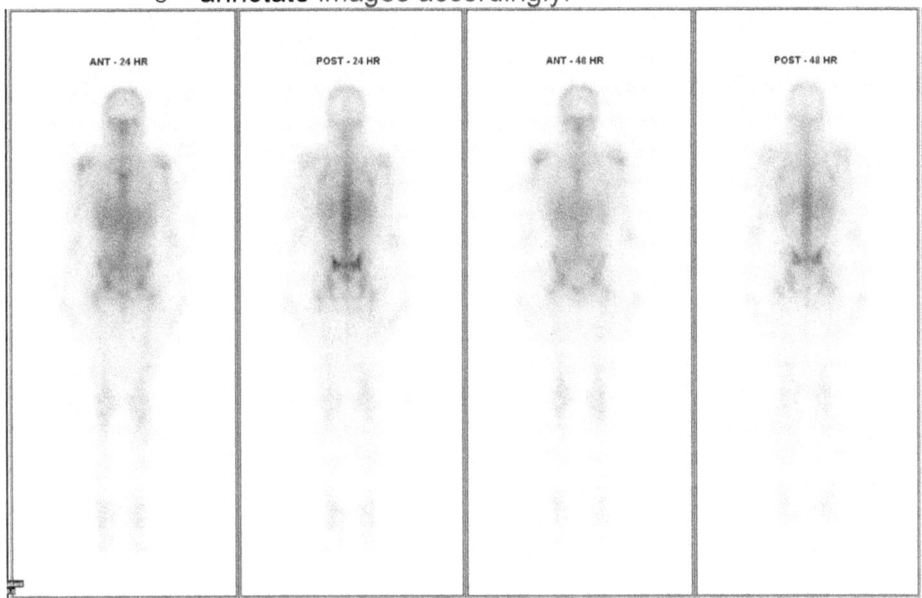

Figure 24 Ga-67 WB 24&48 hours

---

[14] Image processing software used (GE Healthcare Xeleris)

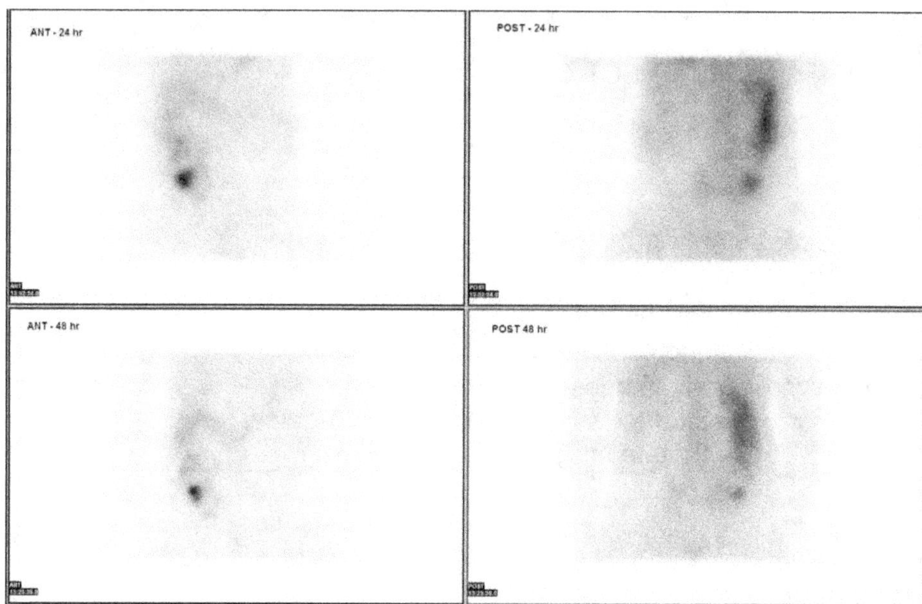

Figure 25 Ga-67 statics 24&48 hours

The first
semester of
the fourth
academic year

السنة الدراسية
الرابعة
الكورس الأول

Fourth Academic Year / First Semester

The subjects that will be studied in this semester are:

1. Nuclear Pharmacy and Radiopharmaceuticals
This subject is divided into theoretical and practical laboratory parts. In the theoretical part, all radioactive materials used in nuclear medicine and patient dose calculation methods are studied. In the practical part, there is a laboratory in one of the nuclear medicine departments, and students are trained in preparing radioactive materials and patient dose preparation. There is a practical test at the end of the semester.

2. Quality Assurance
Measurement of device efficiency (Quality Assurance) and all types of QC used in nuclear medicine are studied in detail.

3. Computer Applications
In this subject, some nuclear medicine examinations previously studied in the Radiographic Procedures subject are revisited, with a focus on the equations used in image processing programs. For example, the kidney scan and the equations used to calculate kidney efficiency will be studied. The exam includes questions similar to the Radiographic Procedures subject with many mathematical problems.

4. Imaging Procedures 3
In the fourth academic year, first semester, the following nuclear medicine examinations are studied:
- Myocardial Perfusion Imaging (MPI)
- Cystography
- Testicular Imaging
- Venography
- Lymph Imaging
- Brain Imaging

In addition to some other topics.

5. Clinical 3
This subject covers the practical part of the examinations studied in the Procedures subject in the fourth academic year, first semester, in addition to what was studied in the third academic year. This means that the practical exam includes all the examinations studied in the third and fourth academic years.

السنة الدراسية الرابعة / الكورس الأول

المواد التي سيتم دراستها في هذا الكورس:

الصيدليه النوويه وعلم الاقربازين
يتم دراسة هذه المادة في جزئين نظري و عملي مختبر .
في الجزء النظري يتم دراسة كافة المواد المشعة المستخدمة في الطب النووي و طرق حساب جرعة المريض.
في الجزء العملي: يكون هناك مختبر في احد اقسام الطب النووي ، و يتدرب الطلبة على تحضير المواد المشعة و تحضير جرعة المريض ، و يكون هناك اختبار عملي في نهاية الفصل.

قياس كفاءة الاجهزة
يتم دراسة كافة انواع ضبطالجودة المستخدمة في الطب النووي بالتفصيل.

استخدام الحاسب الالي فى التصوير الاشعاعى
في هذه المادة يتم دراسة بعض فحوصات الطب النووي التي سبق دراستها في مادة البروسيجر و لكن مع تركيز اكثر على المعادلات المستخدمة في برامج معالجة الصور. على سبيل المثال سوف يتم دراسة فحص الكلى و المعادلات المستخدمة لحساب كفاءة الكلى. الأمتحان يحتوي على اسئلة مشابهة لمادة البروسيجر مع الكثير من المسائل الحسابية.

طرق تصوير اشعاعي 3
في السنة الدراسية الرابعة الكورس الأول يتم دراسة فحص عضلة القلب MPI فقط في كمية الميدتيرم.
و يتم دراسة فحوصات الطب النووي التالية بعد المدتيرم:
Cystography, Testicular Imaging, Venography, Lymph Imaging, Brain Imaging
بالأضافة الى بعض المواضيع الأخرى.

كلينيكال 3
يتم في هذه المادة تغطية الجزء العملي للفحوصات التي يتم دراستها في مادة البروسيجر في السنة الدراسية الرابعة الكورس الأول بالأضافة الى ما تم دراسته في السنة الدراسية الثالثة. أي ان الامتحان العملي يشمل كافة الفحوصات التي تم دراستها في السنة الدراسية الثالثة و الرابعة.

Fourth Academic Year / First Semester Nuclear Medicine Examinations

السنة الدراسية الرابعة / الكورس الأول

فحوصات الطب النووي

1. Myocardial Perfusion Imaging (MPI)
2. Testicular Imaging
3. Lymph Imaging
4. Whole body iodine 131 imaging WBI

Note: The nuclear medicine examination protocols mentioned in this guide are for illustrative purposes only. Please refer to the specific nuclear medicine department for the actual examination protocols in use.

تنويه: بروتكولات فحوصات الطب النووي المذكورة في هذا الدليل هي مجرد مثال توضيحي ، لذا يرجى الرجوع الى بروتكولات فحوصات الطب النووي المستخدمة في قسم الطب النووي الخاص بكم.

1-Myocardial Perfusion Imaging (MPI)

Usually is study is done in two stages stress & rest. CT is done usually with the stress stage and rest is done without CT. In stress stage before the scan the patient should reach a target heart rate ≥85% of maximum predicted heart rate (220-Age), this is done by treadmill exercise or by Pharmacological (the patient is given a medicine like (Dipyridamole (Persentene), Regadosen, Adenosine and Dobutamin). After treadmill exercise the patient is injected with the radiotracer, then given a fatty meal then imaged after 30 minute of injection. After Pharmacological given the patient is injected with the radiotracer, then given a fatty meal then imaged after 60 minute of injection. The fatty meal is given to secrete bilirubin to focus radio tracer on the heart.

Indications

Indications	coronary artery disease.
	Evaluation for coronary bypass surgery

Contraindication:

contraindication	taking chemical stressors (smoke, coffee, soda and chocolate)
	Taking some heart meds

Patient preparation:

Patient preparation	fast 2-6 hour
	Stop (smoke, coffee, soda, chocolate) 24 hour
	stop interfering meds 24-48 hour, bring meds
	men shave chest, ware track suit
	REST scan, only 6 hour fasting, can take all medications

Radiopharmaceutical:

Radiopharmaceutical	T 1/2	Dose	Route of administration	Notes
99mTc-tetrofosmin (MYVIEW)	6 hours- 140 Kev	10-30mci	I.V	half dose 10 mCi
Localization	binds to myocytes			

Equipment:

- Collimator: LEHR or IQ-SMART ZOOM

Views & their parameters:

- Gated TOMO, and CT is done usually with stress scan, not with Rest.

		GE discovery	Siemens Symbia
TOMO	collimator	LEHR	LEHR/ IQ
	matrix	64x64	128x128
	zoom	1.3	1.45
	number of view	60 (120 total)	64-each detector 32
	time per view	20 sec	25 sec
		-IF NO CT 20 sec/f FOR < 85 kg- 25 sec/f < 100 kg- 30 sec/F > 100 kg	
	degree of rotation	90 (90 for each detector total180	90 (90 for each detector total180
	start angle	45-rao-to-lao	45
	detector configuration	90 (90 for each detector total180	90 (90 for each detector total180
	orbit	Non circular (body contour)	NCO Non circular
	mode	step & shoot	step & shoot
	rotation	CCW	CCW

	body contour	on	on
gate	number of frames	8	8
	selected window		30
	center		97 (1-WINDOW-beat/MIN)
	width %		0-on
	Forward/backward by third		0-on
	auto center primary window		0-on
	auto tracking		0-on
	Reject PVC Beats		0-on
	beats to reject post PVC	1	0-on
	PVC threshold	high% - low% 100	200
		if high rejection 125%	
CT	scan type	Helical	
	Voltage	140 keV	130 keV
	Current	2.5 mA	25 mA
	Slice thickness	5 mm	0.6 mm
	pitch	1.9	
	care dose /SMART	0-on	
	use for	AC	
	velocity	2 RPM	
	matrix	512	
	CT RANGE	Partial	

Image processing:

MPI Image processing steps:[15]

- Select the Study, then select Myovation protocol.
- On Recon/Reformat screen, adjust the ROI over the heart.
- Select (Recon / Reformat / Mask) to apply masking.
- Check patient motion on the cined images.
- Adjust reconstruction, reformat limits, and orientation lines.
- Check the gates quality on Gated QC Tap.
- Check the registration quality on Attenuation Correction QC Tap.
- Click review tab.

---

[15] Image processing software used (GE Healthcare Xeleris)

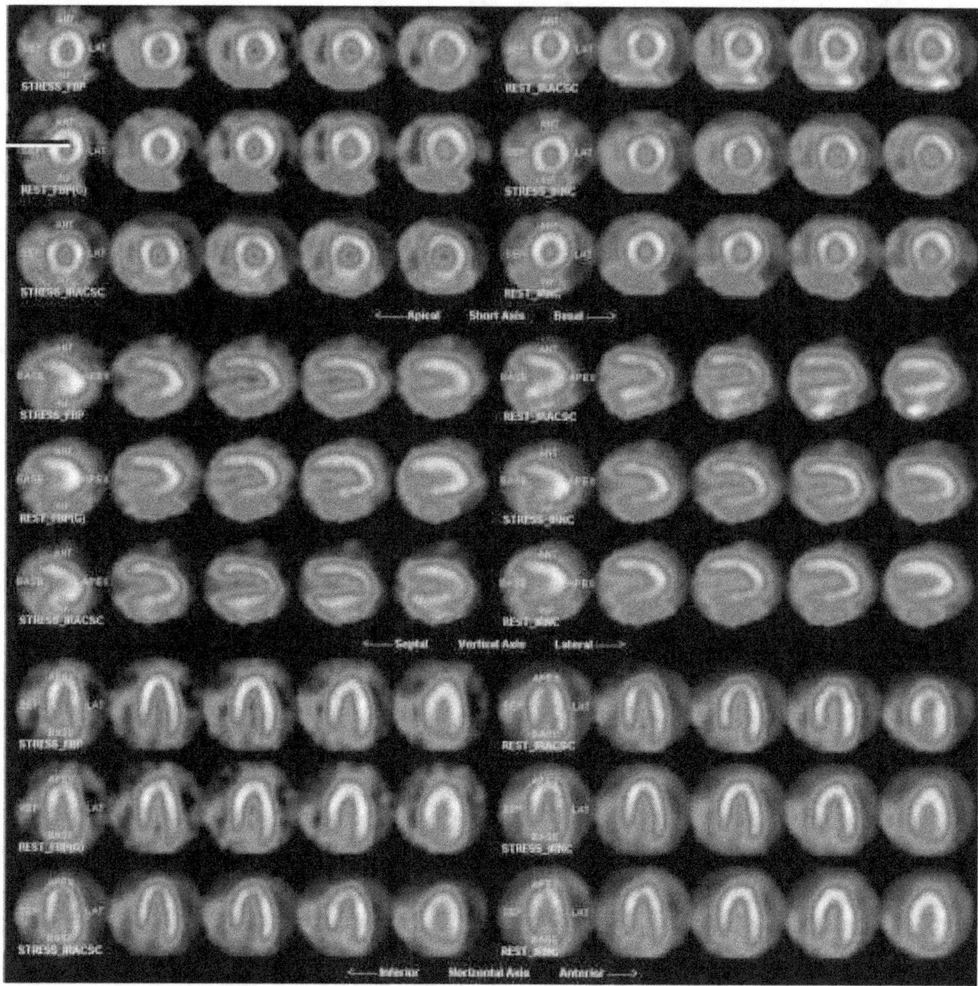

Figure 27 MPI process images

2-Testicular Imaging

Indications

Indications	Differentiation between acute testicular torsion & acute epididymitis
	Evaluation of (groin pain, scrotal mass, & blood supply to testes)

Radiopharmaceutical:

Radiopharmaceutical	T 1/2	Dose	Route of administration
1-Tc-99m pertechnetate	6 hours- 140 Kev	5-15 mCi	I.V
OR 2- DTPA		15 mCi	

Views & their parameters:

1	type	matrix	zoom	time	notes
FLOW	dynamic	128	2	2min	detector 1 anterior
	flow-60F/2sec				
	Tape penis up- sheet under scrotum				

2	type	matrix	zoom	time	notes
STATICS	static	256x256	2	5min each image	detector 1 anterior
	1-BP @ 5min (after flow)				
	2-SPOT @ 10min				
	3-delay				
	4- static with MARKER(on each felt testes or on the raphe of scrotum)				

Image processing:

For processing testicular images, follow these steps:[16]

- Static images:
  - Load the following static images: "immediate," "10 minutes' delay," and "1-hour delay."
  - Annotate the images for the right (RT) and left (LT) testicles.
- Dynamic images:
  - Reframe by 3

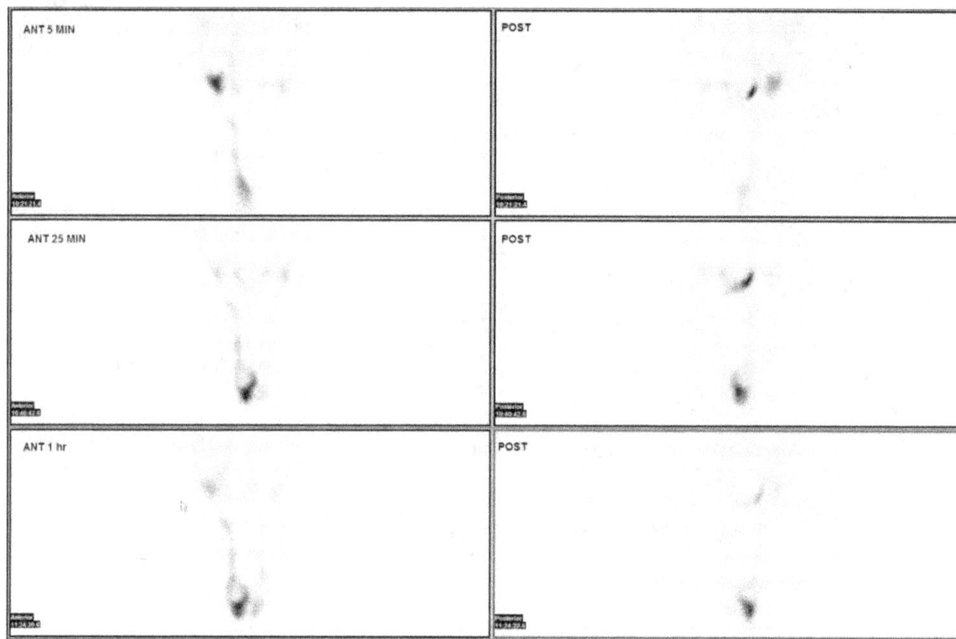

Figure 28 Testicular Statics

3-Lymph Imaging (Upper & Lower Extremities)

Indications

Indications	staging of cancers into the lymph system
	Evaluation of lymphatic drainage for blockage
	lymphedema
	lymph vessel patency

Patient preparation:

Patient preparation	For lymphedema, patient wear elastic stockings. that is removed 3–4 hours before study.
	clean injection area before injection

Radiopharmaceutical:

Radiopharmaceutical	T 1/2	Dose	Route of administration
Tc 99m-SC (NANOCOLLIOD)0r filtered tin colloid	6 hours- 140 Kev	1-1.5	intradermal into the web of hand or foot.
Localization	Compartmental, phagocytosis.		

Views & their parameters:

A-Upper Extremities

	type	matrix	zoom	time	notes
INJECTION SITE	static-	256x256	1	1 min	**FEET FIRST-HEAD OUT**
	injection site feet on center				
	@ 0 MIN				
	@15 MIN				
	@ 30 MIN				
	@60 MIN (1hr)				
	@ 120 MIN (2hr)				

	type	matrix	zoom	SPEED/velocity	notes
WB	static	256x1024	1	10 cm/min	**feet first-head out**
	from injected site to the (liver)-hands over head stretched				
	@ 15 MIN				
	@ 30 MIN				
	@ 60 MIN (1hr) , Include LIVER For QC in 1 hour image				
	@ 120 MIN (2hr)				

B- Lower Extremities

	type	matrix	zoom	time	notes
INJECTION SITE	static	256x256	1	1 min	**HEAD FIRST-FEET out**
	injection site feet on center				
	@ 0 MIN				
	@ 10 MIN				
	@ 60 MIN (1hr)				
	@ 120 MIN (2hr)				
	@ 240 MIN (4hr)				

	type	matrix	zoom	SPEED/velocity	notes
WB	static	256x1024	1	10 cm/min	HEAD FIRST
	from feet to (liver)-lower abdomen				
	@10 MIN				
	@ 60 MIN (1hr) , include LIVER For QC in 1 hour image				
	@ 120 MIN (2hr)				
	@ 240 MIN (4hr)				

Image processing:

For lymphatic system imaging, follow these steps:

- whole-body (WB) images
  - Load all (WB) images for different time points (5 min, 45 min, and 3 hour) and Annotate.
- Static Images
  - Load all static images & Annotate.

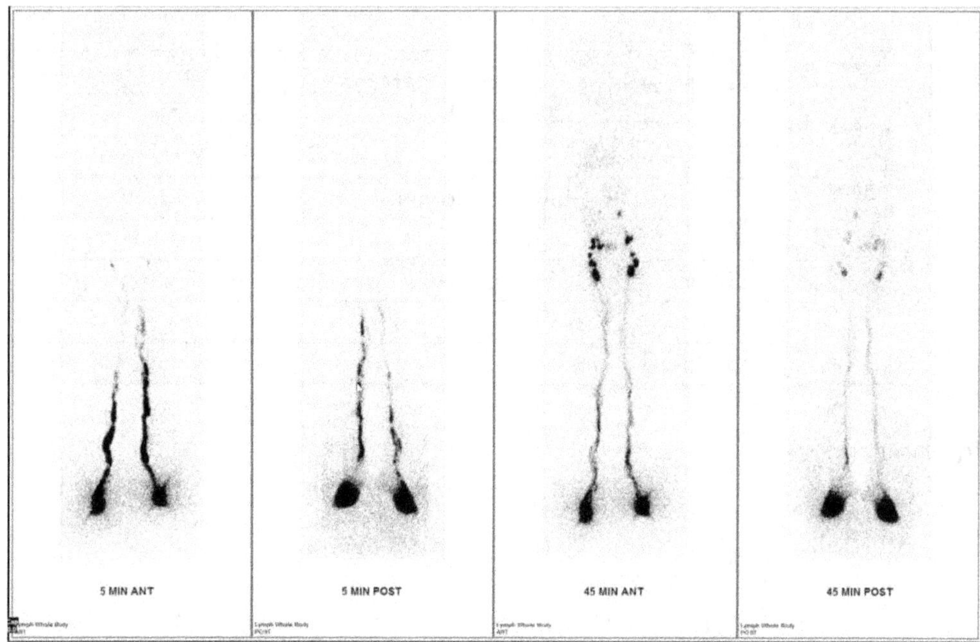

Figure 29 Whole body lower lymph images

4- Whole body iodine 131 imaging WBI

Indications

Indications	detect and localize metastases for thyroid cancer
	post thyroid surgery-thyroidectomy

Contraindication:

contraindication	allergy to iodine if it is used
	pregnant and breast feeding ladies

Patient preparation:

Patient preparation	overnight fasting until 2 hrs post i-131 ingestion
	stop any thyroid medications: thyroxin (T4) for 4-6 weeks- and Cytomel (T3) for 2 weeks
	should not take (thyroid blocking agent) for 5 days before study
	avoid eating iodine containing food. (cabbage-turnips greens-soy beans-shellfish-seafood-kelp-large amount of table salt)

Radiopharmaceutical:

Radiopharmaceutical	T 1/2	Dose	Route of administration
I-131 (sodium iodine)	8 days - 364 Kev	1uci-10mci	131I capsule Oral (PO)
Localization	Active transport.		

Equipment:

- High energy collimator
- Window 20% centered @ 364 Kev

Views & their parameters:

	day 1	day 2	day3,uptake @ 24 hr		day 5-6
protocol	patient given thyrogen 1	pt given thyrogen 2, then given 10-100 uci I131 orally	if < 10% , give 2-3 mci I131	if > 10%, thyroid scan by tc99m	whole body iodine imaging WBI

- No need to be fasting for WB scan, fast only for I131 capsule ingestion before 24hr uptake is done

	type	matrix	zoom
WB	Static	256x1024	1
	scan length 130, because thyroid Ca rarely goes under knees		
	scan speed 6		
	start from top of head to knees		

- SPECT-CT Then is done over neck and chest area.

Image processing:

For WB I-131 imaging, follow these steps:
- whole-body (WB) images
  - Load all (WB) images and Annotate.
- SPECT-CT Images
  - Select Tomo and Ct, then select Volimitrix protocol.

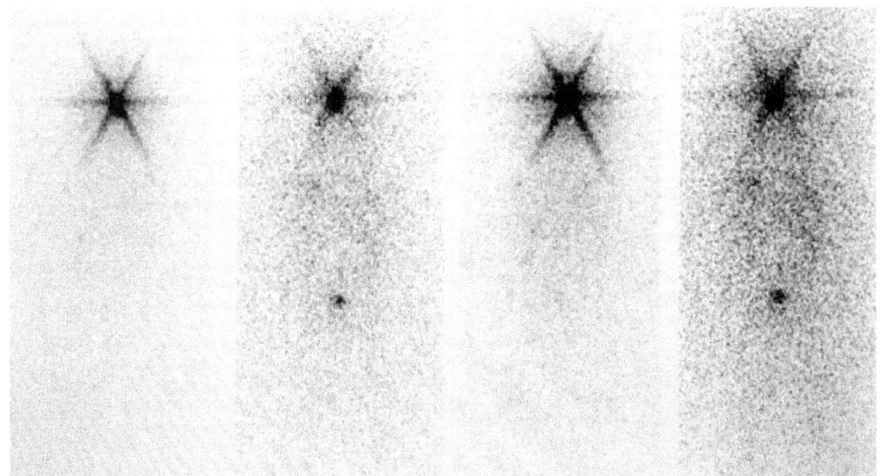

Figure 30 I131-wb images

The second semester of the fourth academic year

السنة الدراسية الرابعة الكورس الثاني

Fourth Academic Year / Second Semester

The subjects that will be studied in this semester are:

1. Nuclear Medicine and Pathology of Blood Diseases (haematology)

This subject is divided into theoretical and practical laboratory parts. In the theoretical part, nuclear medicine examinations that rely on studying the patient's blood are studied. In the practical part, there is a laboratory in one of the nuclear medicine departments where students are trained in these studies and In-Vitro Studies (laboratory test methods). There is a practical test at the end of the semester.

2. Research

During lectures, students will initiate research that will culminate in writing a final research report. The graduation research is done in groups, and one of the college professors is responsible for each group. The college professor supervises the completion of the research, assists students in choosing the research topic and its methodology, and helps solve problems that students encounter during the research. At the end of the semester, students submit the final research report and make a presentation where each group explains the research they conducted. There is also a research poster that is displayed on the day of the scientific poster presentation, where the best scientific research is announced.

3. Pathology in Imaging

In this subject, various diseases are studied.

4. Imaging Procedures 4

In the fourth academic year, second semester, the following nuclear medicine examinations are studied:
- PET Imaging
- Le Veen Shunt Imaging
- Dacro Imaging
- Salivary Imaging
- Somatostatin Receptor Imaging
- Monoclonal Antibody Imaging
- Mammogram Imaging

In addition to some other topics.

5. Clinical 4

This subject covers the practical part of the examinations that are studied in the Procedures subject in the fourth academic year, second semester, in addition to what was studied in the previous semester and the third academic year. It's important to note that usually PET Imaging is typically covered in the Procedures subject and is not included in the practical exam.

السنة الدراسية الرابعة / الكورس الثاني

المواد التي سيتم دراستها في هذا الكورس:

طرق الفحوصات المختبريه

. يتم دراسة هذه المادة في جزئين نظري و عملي مختبر

في الجزء النظري يتم دراسة علم الدم و امراضه في الطب النووي و فحوصات الطب النووي التي تعتمد على دراسة دم المريض .

في الجزء العملي: يكون هناك مختبر في احد اقسام الطب النووي ، و يتدرب الطلبة على هذه الدراسات ، و يكون هناك اختبار عملي في نهاية الفصل.

بحث

في محاضرات مادة بحث التخرج يتم شرح خطوات كتابة البحث بالتدرج ابتداء من اختيار عنوان البحث و انتهاءا بكتابة تقرير البحث النهائي.

لأجراء بحث التخرج يقسم الطلبة الى مجموعات و يكون مسئول عن كل مجموعة احد اساتذة الكلية ، يشرف استاذ الكلية المسئول عن المجموعة على اتمام البحث و يساعد الطلبة على اختيار موضوع البحث و طريقة اجرائه و يسهم في حل المشاكل التي تواجه الطلبة اثناء القيام بالبحث.

في نهاية الفصل يقوم الطلبة بتسليم تقرير البحث النهائي ، و كذلك يقومون بعمل عرض تقديمي ، تشرح فيه كل مجموعة البحث الذي اجرته ، و كذلك يقومون بعمل بوستر البحث الذي يتم عرضه في يوم الملصق العلمي الذي يتم فيه اعلان افضل بحث علمي.

علم الامراض التصويرى (٢)

في هذه المادة يتم دراسةالعديد من الأمرض.

طرق تصوير اشعاعي 4

في السنة الدراسية الرابعة الكورس الثاني يتم دراسة (PET imaging) و بعد الميدترم يتم دراسة الفحوصات التالية:

Le Veen Shunt imaging, Dacro imaging, Salivary imaging, somatostatin Receptor imaging, Monoclonal antibody imaging, Mammogram imaging

بالأضافة الى بعض المواضيع الأخرى.

كلينيكال 4

يتم في هذه المادة تغطية الجزء العملي للفحوصات التي يتم دراستها في مادة البروسيجر في السنة الدراسية الرابعة الكورس الثاني بالأضافة الى ما تم دراسته في الكورس السابق و السنة الدراسية الثالثة. أي ان الامتحان العملي يشمل كافة الفحوصات التي تم دراستها في السنة الدراسية الثالثة و الرابعة.

ملاحظة: غالبا يتم تغطية PET imaging في مادة البروسيجر ولا يتم تغطيته في الامتحان العملي (الكلينيكال).

السنة الدراسية الرابعة / الكورس الثاني

فحوصات الطب النووي

Fourth Academic Year / Second Semester Nuclear Medicine Examinations

1. (Lacrimal Study) Dacryo scintigraphy
2. Salivary Gland Imaging

Note: The nuclear medicine examination protocols mentioned in this guide are for illustrative purposes only. Please refer to the specific nuclear medicine department for the actual examination protocols in use.

تنويه: بروتكولات فحوصات الطب النووي المذكورة في هذا الدليل هي مجرد مثال توضيحي ، لذا يرجى الرجوع الى بروتكولات فحوصات الطب النووي المستخدمة في قسم الطب النووي الخاص بكم.

1- (Lacrimal Study) Dacryo scintigraphy

Indications

Indications	lacrimal duct patency
	nasolacrimal duct obstruction
	epiphora

Radiopharmaceutical:

Radiotracer	T 1/2	Dose	Route of administration
1-Tc-99m pertechnetate	6 hours- 140 Kev	50–200 uCi	eye-dropper

Equipment:

- Collimator LEHR or Pinhole

Views & their parameters:

1	type	matrix	zoom	Phase
DYNAMIC	dynamic	128	2	45 frames / 20 sec each
	radiotracer given by eye dropper on patient eyes while patient laying			
	After 5 min dynamic image taken while patient standing or setting			
	Patient face in front of detector			

2	type	matrix	zoom	time	notes
STATICS	static	256	2	5 min	Patient face to detector
	15 minute				
	20minute				
	30 minute				
	60 minute				

Image processing:

For processing Lacrimal (Dacryoscintigraphy) images, follow these steps:

- Statics:
    - Load all the static images (15 min, 20 min, 30 min, 60 min) to a new workspace.
    - Annotate the static images.
- Dynamic Images:
    - Load all the dynamic images.
    - Choose a layout of 5x3 for dynamic images.
    - Set the dynamic frame rate to 1 minute/frame

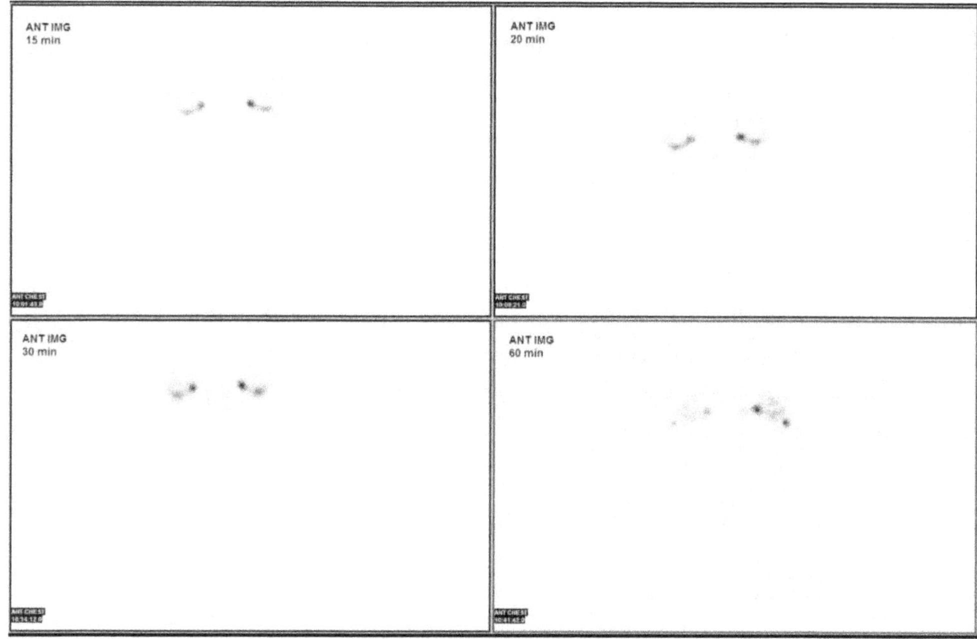

Figure 31 Lacrimal static images

2- Salivary Gland Imaging

Indications

Indications	Evaluation of salivary gland function, size and position
	salivary duct obstruction
	salivary gland mass and tumors

Patient preparation:

Patient preparation	stop thyroid-blocking agents for 48 hours before exam.
	give gum or citrus-flavored candy to stimulate salivary glands.

Radiopharmaceutical:

Radiotracer	T 1/2	Dose	Route of administration
1-Tc-99m pertechnetate	6 hours- 140 Kev	8-12 mCi	I.V

Views & their parameters:

1	type	matrix	time	notes
DYNAMIC	dynamic	128	30 min	Anterior
	flow 60 frames / 1 sec each			
	Dynamic 60 frames / 30 sec each			

2	type	matrix	zoom	time	count-Kcount	notes
STATIC	static-	256	1.23	180 sec	Or 300	Anterior
	1- Anterior					
	2- R LAT/ L LAT					

Image processing:

For processing Salivary Gland images, follow these steps:

- Statics:
    - Load all the static images & Annotate.
- Dynamic Images:
    - Load the dynamic images.
    - Draw ROI over salivary glands and generate Time-Activity-Curve.

Nuclear Medicine Clinical Procedures for Technologists

References

- Nuclear Medicine Technology: Procedures and Quick Reference, Second Edition, Pete Shackett.

- The examination protocols for nuclear medicine described in this manual are derived from my experiences as a nuclear medicine technology student during the third and fourth academic years (2019/2017) at several nuclear medicine departments, including:
    o Nuclear Medicine Department at Ibn Sina Hospital - Hamed Al-Essa Organ Transplant Center, Kuwait.
    o Nuclear Medicine Department at Chest Hospital, Kuwait.
    o Nuclear Medicine Department at Kuwait Cancer Control Center, Kuwait.
    o Nuclear Medicine Department at Mubarak Al-Kabeer Hospital, Kuwait.
    o Nuclear Medicine Department at Amiri Hospital, Kuwait.

OTHER AUTHOR PUBLICATIONS

109

- Nuclear Medicine Hot Lab for Technologists

- CT in Nuclear Medicine.

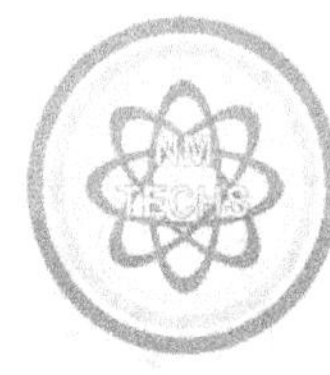

NM Techs™

Educational Recourses for Nuclear Medicine Technologists

Telegram:	NM_Techs
YouTube:	NM_Techs
Twitter:	Nm_Techs
Instagram:	nm_techs
Facebook:	NM Techs
Threads:	nm_techs
Email:	nm.techs.kh@gmail.com

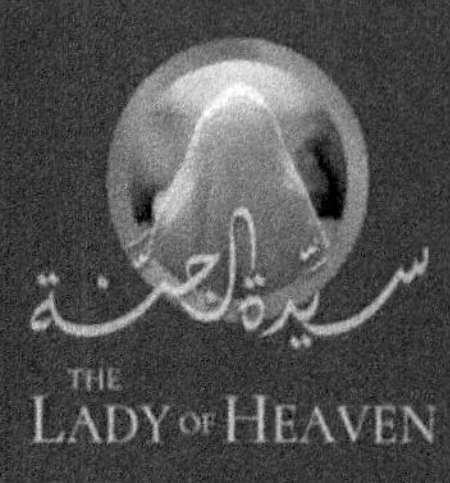

ماذا على من شمّ تربة أحمد أن لا يشمّ مدى الزّمان غواليا
صبّت عليّ مصائب لو أنّها صبّت على الأيّام صرن لياليا
قل للمغيّب تحت أطباق الثّرى إن كنت تسمع صرختي وندائيا
قد كنت ذات حمى بظلّ محمّد لا أخش من ضيم وكان جماليا
فاليوم أخضع للذّليل وأتّقي ضيمي وأدفع ظالمي بردائيا
فاذا بكت قمريّة في ليلها شجنا على غصن بكيت صباحيا
فلأجعلنّ الحزن بعدك مونسـي ولأجعلنّ الدّمع فيك وشاحيا

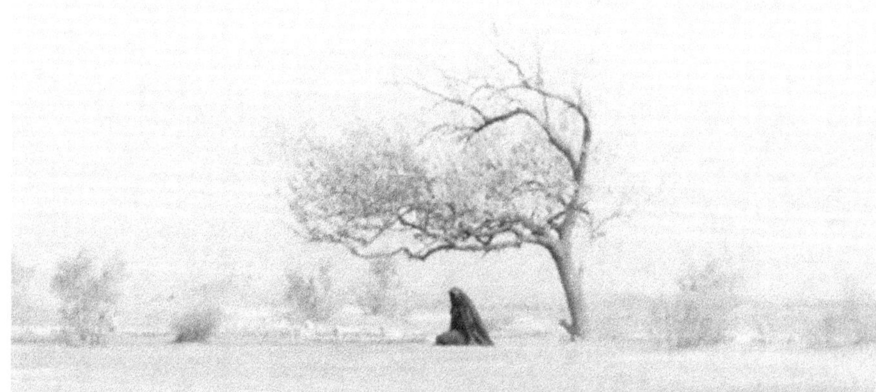